10655832

DR. COHEN'S HEALTHY SAILOR BOOK

Michael Martin Cohen, M.D.

DR. COHEN'S HEALTHY SAILOR BOOK

 Patrick Stephens, Cambridge

© 1983 by International Marine Publishing Company

All rights reserved. Except for use in a review, no part of this book may be reproduced or utilized in any form or by any means, electronic or mechanical, including photocopying, recording, or by any information storage and retrieval system, without written permission from Patrick Stephens Limited.

First published in the United States of America 1983 by International Marine Publishing Company.

This edition published in the United Kingdom 1984 by Patrick Stephens Limited, Bar Hill, Cambridge, CB3 8EL, England

Printed and bound in the United States of America

ISBN 0-85059-715-3

for Elisse and Jordan

Contents

Preface

SAILORS BY NATURE AND necessity are a self-sufficient lot. They often
acquire a considerable amount of technical information, ranging from
the sublime science of celestial navigation to the nuts-and-bolts mechanics
of the marine engine. And yet, the one machine upon which the sailor
ultimately depends—the human body—remains largely a mystery.

The aim of this book is not first aid. There are plenty of first-aid books
available. Rather, it was conceived as a guide to health on the water. Its
purpose is to cut through the mystery and explore the ways in which the
human body functions (and malfunctions) in a nautical environment. The
premise is that if the sailor understands the particular stresses he is likely
to encounter at sea, he will be able to *anticipate* and *avoid* potential prob-

lems and keep himself and his crew members healthy and happy. In the process he will inevitably discard many of the accumulated misconceptions and old wives' tales that characterize the nautical-medicine tradition. Finally, the sailor will be able to evaluate critically the sailing fads and fallacies that arise from time to time.

I would like to thank my many friends and colleagues who have assisted in the preparation of this book. They include Robert F. Russell, M.D.; Robert S. Pratt; Pedro Fernandez, M.D.; Bernard A. Kirshbaum, M.D.; Joni Youngwirth; Nelson M. Wolf, M.D.; Oksana M. Korzeniowski, M.D.; Stephen A. Youngwirth, M.D.; Simmons Lessell, M.D.; Carl E. Klafs, Ph.D.; James C. Sattel; Edward R. Cohen; Trudy Cohen; Laverne C. Johnson, Ph.D.; Elliot D. Weitzman, M.D.; T. H. Monk, Ph.D.; and Stephen C. Mann, M.D. Samuel S. Cohen deserves special acknowledgment for his invaluable comments and criticisms. Finally, without the support, understanding, and advice of my wife, Elisse Reidbord Cohen, Ph.D., this book could never have been completed.

DR. COHEN'S HEALTHY SAILOR BOOK

1

Seasickness

And I'm never, never sick at sea!
What, never?
No, never!
What, never?
Well, hardly ever!
He's hardly ever sick at sea!
Then give three cheers, and one cheer more
For the hardy Captain of the Pinafore!

W. S. Gilbert, *HMS Pinafore*, 1878

ACCORDING TO AN ENGLISH sailors' proverb, "The only cure for seasickness is to sit on the shady side of an old brick church in the country." Despite its obvious facetiousness, this proverb highlights a frequently overlooked fact, namely, that seasickness is a disorder we inflict upon ourselves! Seasickness did not exist until our ancestors relinquished the relative security of land for the uncertainty of a raft or canoe. Written accounts date back at least as far as the ancient Greeks. Hippocrates wrote, "Sailing on the sea proves that motion disturbs the body," a statement that contains more insight and less misconjecture than most of what was written during the next 2,000 years! Our English word *nausea* is, in fact, derived from the Greek word *naus,* which means ship.

1

Because of our long familiarity with seasickness, numerous misconceptions and old wives' tales surround the illness. Nevertheless, we have made major advances in our understanding of both its causes and treatment. The first advance (in the 19th century) was the awareness that motion is the cause of *motion sickness* and that seasickness is simply one form of motion sickness (essentially Hippocrates' discovery). Riding in cars, trains, airplanes, spacecraft, and on elephants and camels produces the same symptoms! Lawrence of Arabia, for example, suffered from "camel sickness"—a doubly appropriate term since camels are the "ships of the desert." More recently, about 30 percent of the astronauts and cosmonauts who have flown in space have experienced motion sickness, or "spacecraft sickness."

When man depended on *active locomotion* —his own two feet—to get around, there was no problem. Running, jumping, somersaulting, and other such activities do not usually cause motion sickness. Only with the advent of *passive locomotion* (initially sailing and the riding of some domesticated animals) did motion sickness appear. We may find some consolation in noting that most other animal species are also liable to motion sickness when subjected to passive locomotion, including birds, dogs, horses, sheep, pigs, and even fish! Of all the species that have been tested so far, only rabbits and guinea pigs seem to be immune. The fact that motion sickness affects so many different species tells us something about the region of the brain that is responsible. It is not the more recently evolved portion—the cerebral hemispheres—that controls motion sickness, but rather the older, more primitive hindbrain, which we share with many other animal species. The function of the hindbrain is discussed in more detail later in this chapter.

The next advance was the recognition that motion sickness is a disorder of the brain and not of the stomach. Previous studies were mainly concerned with the stomach, which explains the variety of diets that have been proposed for the embarking passenger as well as for those already in the throes of seasickness. A popular theory in the last century attributed seasickness to the shifting of the stomach and intestines. Devices were invented that could be worn around the middle to restrict this motion. Someone even recommended that the passenger "should wear a pad in the epigastrium [abdomen] with an opposing one in the small of the back, and, at the first qualms, should cause a mild galvanic current to pass between the two." Speculation that the inner ear and its connections with the brain were the source of motion sickness did not begin until the 1880s, and there were doubting Thomases well into the 20th century.

The third advance we have yet to make. We still do not know the precise area of the brain responsible for seasickness or why nausea and vomiting occur (as opposed to some other symptom such as coughing, sneezing, or hiccups).

Most of the recent research has centered on two aspects of the problem: the types of motion that cause motion sickness and the means of prevention. For the sailor, they are the major concerns. First, however, it is necessary to understand the operation of the balance mechanism itself. Unless the sailor knows the basics of this system, he will be "at sea" when confronted with some of the outrageous forms of treatment that are proposed from time to time.

THE VESTIBULAR (BALANCE) SYSTEM

There are three parts to the inner ear: the *cochlea,* or hearing apparatus, the *semicircular canals,* and the *utricle* and *saccule* (U&S) (Figure 1.1). Since these structures are embedded in the skull, they move *pari passu* with movements of the head; that is, if the head is moved up or down or to the right or left, these structures move exactly the same amount. The implication will soon become clear.

The utricle and saccule developed first, and their major task is relatively straightforward—determining the direction of gravity (i.e., telling up from down). Both the utricle and the saccule consist of an array of hair cells upon which is balanced a solid mass of calcium carbonate crystals embedded in a gelatinous matrix (Figure 1.2*A*). The entire structure is bathed in a watery fluid called *endolymph.* Since the crystalline-gelatinous matrix is three times as dense as the endolymph, when the head is tilted away from the vertical position, gravity attracts the matrix (Figure 1.2*B*). As the matrix shifts, the hair cells are bent, producing a change in the number of nerve impulses relayed to the brain. The U&S function identically, except that in the utricle the hair cells are oriented horizontally and in the saccule, vertically.

Although the U&S developed as gravity detectors, they also register *linear acceleration:* movement forward or backward, right or left, and up or down. Actually, gravity *is* a form of linear acceleration with a constant value of 32 feet per second per second and a constant direction, perpendicular to the earth. The key to understanding this dual function of gravity orientation and linear acceleration is *inertia.* The law of inertia states that any mass at rest tends to remain at rest and any mass in motion tends to remain in motion unless acted upon by an outside force.

With this in mind, let us look at what happens during a common

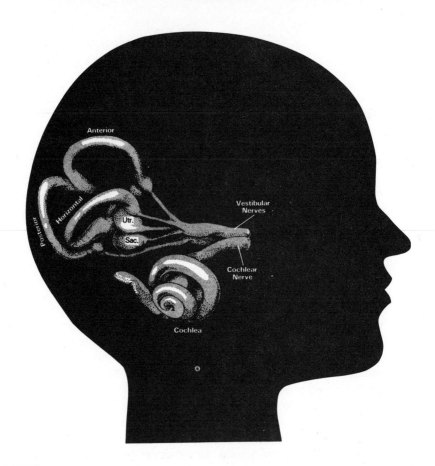

Figure 1.1. The vestibular (balance) system.

experience—forward acceleration in a car. As we accelerate, the U&S also accelerate forward—except, that is, the crystalline-gelatinous matrix that lies upon the hair cells. Because of inertia, the matrix is temporarily "left behind." Again, the hair cells are bent, this time signaling forward linear acceleration (Figure 1.2C).

Usually there is no confusion as to whether we are experiencing head tilt or forward acceleration. After all, we can *feel* our body being thrust backward (inertia again), and we can *see* that we are moving forward. In other words, *we place the information in context with the information our other senses provide.* When we are deprived of our other senses, especially vision, it may be impossible to tell the difference. This presents a continual hazard for pilots who fly without instruments during periods of reduced visibility. Deprived of visual cues, the pilot may misinterpret rapid forward acceleration as backward head tilt; backward head tilt is,

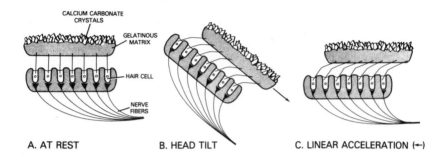

CALCIUM CARBONATE CRYSTALS

GELATINOUS MATRIX

HAIR CELL

NERVE FIBERS

A. AT REST   B. HEAD TILT   C. LINEAR ACCELERATION (←)

Figure 1.2. The utricle and saccule.

after all, more common. Because the pilot has the illusion that he has been gaining altitude, when in fact he has not, he may level off the plane prematurely, producing a nose dive with disastrous consequences.

The U&S function well up to a point, but to allow a greater degree of movement, a more sophisticated device is needed: the semicircular canals, which measure *rotatory acceleration.* There are three semicircular canals on each side of the head: the horizontal (which is actually slightly tilted), the anterior, and the posterior (Figure 1.1). The canals are perpendicular to one another so that all three dimensions of space can be analyzed without gaps in the coverage. Each canal is a small, circular, unbroken tube filled with endolymph. At one point in each canal there is a swelling that contains the *cupula,* a jellylike, elastic structure (Figure 1.3*A*). The cupula protrudes into the tube much like a swinging door and, like a swinging door, it can bend to either side; but at rest, it tends to remain in a neutral position. The cupula has no independent motion. Rather, it is passively displaced by the endolymph in the canal.

To ensure that the canals *do not* respond to gravity, nature employed a cunning stratagem by reducing the density of the cupula until it was exactly the same as the surrounding endolymph. If the cupula were either lighter or heavier, it would bend with head tilting. Since it is the same density, head tilting has no effect.

Embedded in the base of the cupula are numerous hair cells. If the moving endolymph displaces the cupula in one direction, the hair cells are stimulated; if in the opposite direction, they are inhibited.

What happens when we rotate our head to the left? Since the move-

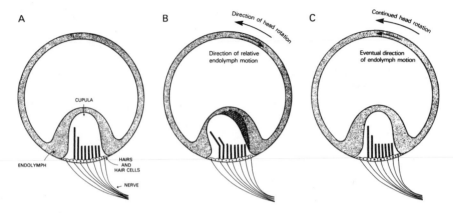

Figure 1.3. The semicircular canals.

ment is restricted to the horizontal plane, only the horizontal canals are involved. The left horizontal canal is rotated to the left by the same amount, say, 20 degrees, since it is embedded in the skull. But the endolymph tends to remain at rest because of inertia. Thus, *relative to the canal,* the endolymph is moving in the opposite direction, to the right (Figure 1.3*B*). This relative motion of the endolymph bends the cupula, which stimulates the hair and nerve cells. Each canal is paired with one on the opposite side with which it works in tandem. If one canal is stimulated, its mate is inhibited. During a leftward head rotation, for example, the right horizontal canal is inhibited. These same concepts apply to nonhorizontal head movements, except that more than one set of canals is involved. Various combinations of canals provide the brain with very precise information regarding rotation of the head and body.

CURRENT THEORIES OF MOTION SICKNESS

In order to maintain balance, even on terra firma, we are endowed with three interrelated systems. The most important is the *vestibular system.* In fact, a functioning vestibular system is a sine qua non to experiencing motion sickness. Most people who have a deficient vestibular system have one consolation—they will not suffer from motion sickness. In the 1880s, it was discovered that most deaf-mutes were immune to seasickness and other forms of motion sickness. Since most of the diseases that produced deafness in that era (e.g., scarlet fever) also affected the vestibular system,

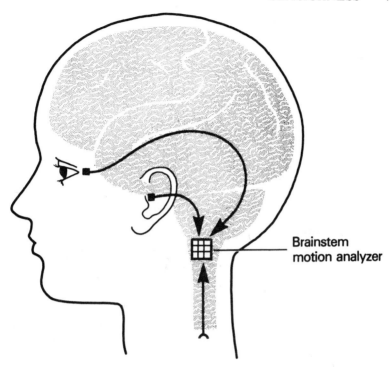

Figure 1.4. The motion analyzer.

this evidence was the first to implicate the vestibular system in motion sickness.

The second system is *vision*. Visual information supplements the information that the vestibular system provides. If we trip over a curbstone and fall forward, not only does our vestibular system signal the fall, but also we *see* that earth and nose are about to enjoy an unwanted familiarity. On occasion the visual system can "override" the information that the vestibular system gives us. Ice skaters, for example, use visual cues to help prevent dizziness when spinning. They learn to rely on the visual signals and suppress the unwanted vestibular signals.

The third system consists of *position sensors* in the joints and tendons of the neck, which signal movement of the head on the body.

All of this information is precisely integrated and analyzed in the hindbrain in a structure we can call the motion analyzer (Figure 1.4). The motion analyzer is composed of nerve cells that respond to signals from all three systems. It processes the data and rapidly arrives at a meaningful response—a kind of computer, if you will.

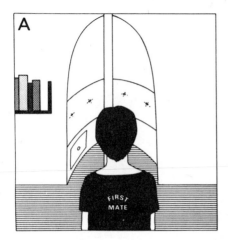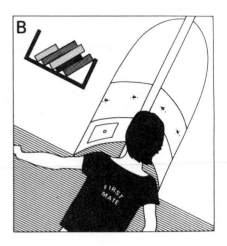

Figure 1.5. Rolling motion to starboard with visual-vestibular conflict.

With three systems providing similar information, there is built-in redundancy. Redundancy is generally a desirable design feature of a system. The advantages are obvious. If one component of the system fails, everything doesn't grind to a halt. With regard to motion, redundancy is both a blessing and a curse. In health it is a blessing, because it provides more sources of information, allowing smooth, coordinated movement. And even if disease should affect one of the systems (e.g., blindness or inner ear disorders), the other two can take up the slack. Redundancy becomes a curse, however, when the three systems are at variance with one another. A conflict in the information these three sources provide the brain produces motion sickness.

This conflict explains why seasickness frequently occurs or is exacerbated by going below decks. Let us suppose that a crew member is seated at the navigation table facing forward during a rolling motion to starboard. The vestibular system senses this movement and duly informs the brain. However, since the hull of the boat has rolled to starboard by the same amount as the navigator, there is no significant change in what the navigator sees (Figure 1.5). The visual system informs the brain that nothing has changed. The brain's motion analyzer has clearly received two sets of conflicting information. If, in addition, the head should jerk forward-backward or side-to-side on the body, a third set of erroneous information is provided. Actually, these extra, involuntary head movements seem to be very important in producing seasickness. As we

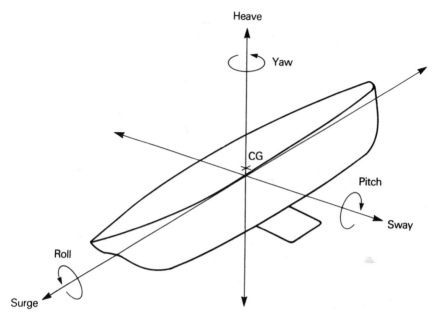

Figure 1.6. *The six motions of a boat: three rotatory (roll, pitch, and yaw) and three linear (surge, heave, and sway).*

will see, reducing them by stabilizing the head tends to ameliorate the seasickness.

As if this is not enough, the brain must deal with yet another set of conflicting information arising from within the vestibular system itself. Normally, the semicircular canals and U&S act as complements, which they have been doing since they first appeared in fish over a million years ago! However, in a rough sea the vestibular system is stimulated in a chaotic fashion. In response to waves, a boat (as well as its crew) is subjected to six different motions: three rotatory (roll, pitch, and yaw), which primarily stimulate the canals, and three linear (surge, heave, and sway), which primarily stimulate the U&S (Figure 1.6). Combined rotatory and linear motions, such as pitching plus heaving or rolling plus surging, *or* rotations about two or more axes simultaneously, such as rolling plus pitching or pitching plus yawing, are very effective in producing seasickness. These complex motions trigger the release of conflicting and irreconcilable sensory information from within the semicircular canals and the U&S.[1]

Any theory of seasickness (and of the other forms of motion sickness) should explain the three phases of the disorder. In this regard, the overstimulation theory is deficient. The first phase, the seasickness itself, *could* be explained by overstimulation of the vestibular system. Following prolonged stimulation during the first phase, the brain's motion analyzer creates a modus vivendi, and the symptoms decline and disappear. Even this second stage, adaptation, could be explained by overstimulation; i.e., in the face of continued stimulation, the canals and/or U&S might be temporarily worn out. However, the third phase is inexplicable by the overstimulation theory. This phase has been termed *mal de debarquement,* the sickness the sailor experiences on stepping ashore after recovering from a bout of seasickness (*mal de mer*). If the term *sea legs* connotes the ability to walk around a boat without experiencing sickness or disequilibrium, then perhaps *land legs* would be an appropriate term for the ability to adjust quickly to land. Why should a sailor become sick all over again when he steps ashore? Clearly it is not due to overstimulation of the vestibular system, since the sailor has now returned to his normal terrestrial environment.

The most appealing explanation is that there is a conflict in the sensory information the brain receives, as described above. According to this theory, which J. T. Reason, J. J. Brand, and others have proposed, the motion analyzer eventually adjusts to the conflict by *rearranging* the sensory information.[2] When the sailor is exposed to a situation that generates sensory conflict, whether among the vestibular, visual, and neck position systems *or* within the vestibular system *or* both, the motion analyzer searches its "memory" for previous similar episodes. If it finds a strong memory trace of sensory conflict comparable to the present situation, nothing happens. If it finds nothing appropriate, it does two things. First, it sets into motion the seasickness syndrome. Why this occurs, we do not know. Next, it begins to fill its memory bank with this new conflicting information (rolls plus heaves, yaws plus surges, and so forth). With time, this conflicting information becomes the norm, and the motion analyzer eventually can search its memory and state categorically, "Yes, I am aware that this combination of sensory information may seem peculiar, but for this environment, which is my home at the present time, it is perfectly OK." This sensory rearrangement coincides with the second, or adaptation, phase; it is a form of unconscious learning. The adaptation phase occurs only if the sailor *continues to be exposed to the same abnormal motion.*

However, when the sailor, who has finally adapted, returns to a terrestrial environment, the motion analyzer is again nonplussed. It searches its memory and on superficial perusal discovers that once again there is a conflict. The motion analyzer has come to expect the unusual combinations of movement.

Again it sets into motion the seasickness syndrome (now mal de debarquement) and searches through its memory more thoroughly. It soon discovers that this particular environment is not so foreign after all. Here we have the crucial difference between mal de mer and mal de debarquement. In the first instance, the process of sensory rearrangement or learning takes an appreciable amount of time to occur, during which the seasickness prevails; whereas in the second instance, the memory has been there all along, merely concealed beneath the more recent information. For this reason, mal de debarquement is never as prolonged as the original episode of seasickness.

SYMPTOMS AND SIGNS

With all of this conflicting information, it may seem surprising that the brain does not rebel more often. Well, it probably does! We undoubtedly underestimate the incidence of seasickness by concentrating on the nausea, vomiting, and "dry heaves." We tend to neglect the earlier "head" symptoms and signs, such as skin pallor, cold sweating, headache, malaise, and dizziness (Table 1.1). These symptoms are frequently attributed to such things as fatigue, anxiety, or dietary indiscretions. Recognition of these signs is important. It is the last opportunity to modify the syndrome to any significant degree before "all hell breaks loose."

The most consistent early sign of seasickness is skin pallor. It invariably precedes other symptoms and signs, but may be easily overlooked in the Sturm und Drang of heavy weather conditions. Cold sweating is next in appearance, but is a less reliable symptom. Headache is common during the early stage. It tends to be mild, usually a dull aching over the eyes or a bandlike constriction around the head. By this time the sailor may feel somewhat drowsy and begin to lose interest in his surroundings and in food. Although he does not as yet have nausea or stomach pain, the sailor becomes increasingly aware of his stomach region. This heightened stomach awareness then blends imperceptibly into queasiness and nausea.

Up to this point, if the abnormal motion ceases, the seasickness abates and the sailor rapidly recovers a sense of well-being. If the stimulus continues, the major manifestations of nausea and vomiting usually occur. The Rubicon has been crossed. The syndrome now takes on a life of its own and, even if the stimulus moderates, the symptoms may endure for an appreciable period of time.

Nausea and vomiting are not invariably linked to one another; some people vomit without premonitory nausea, whereas others experience intense nausea but never vomit. Many individuals find some relief after a bout of vomiting, that is, until a fresh wave of nausea and vomiting occurs.

TABLE 1.1
Common Symptoms and Signs

Head Symptoms
Skin Pallor
Cold Sweating
Headache
Malaise
Dizziness
Drowsiness
Yawning and Sighing
Hyperventilation
Increased Salivation or Dry Mouth

Gut Symptoms
Disinclination to Eat
Stomach Awareness
Queasiness
Nausea
Vomiting or Dry Heaves

Because intense nausea and vomiting (or the dry heaves) are so conspicuous, there is a tendency to equate them with seasickness. This is not correct, however. Some individuals have little or no nausea or vomiting, but are nonetheless more uncomfortable than their mates draped over the leeward rail. Those with predominantly "head" symptoms mope about the deck preferring to be left alone. When this torpid state becomes extreme, it resembles a severe depression, and its sufferers "occasionally beg to be thrown overboard, as life has lost all its charm." Performance of duty may be more hampered in these individuals than in crew members who are vomiting intermittently.

Whether or not a person develops seasickness depends primarily on two factors: (1) the sea conditions and (2) individual susceptibility. If the sea conditions are severe enough, even the most iron-gutted sailor may become sick (assuming that he has a functioning vestibular system). Some evidence suggests that heading directly into the wave system is the point of sailing most likely to cause seasickness. In this situation it is impossible to avoid the combination of multiple rotatory and linear motions described earlier in this chapter.

The experience of K. Adlard Coles is worth examining. In his classic text *Heavy Weather Sailing,* he refers to numerous encounters with gale-force and near-gale-force conditions, but only twice does he give explicit descriptions of seasickness.

One episode occurred while crossing the English Channel during a race.

> By dawn on Sunday (8 August) the wind had moderated, but in *Cohoe*'s cabin conditions did not seem much quieter. For a while after a gale the sea is often more truculent than during its height. The yacht is no longer steadied by the wind and the motion is worse in consequence. At 0700 I got up. I felt amazingly well and refreshed, for I had had a good deal of sleep—more than we got at any other time in the race. I went forward through the cabin and tried the radio, as we wanted a weather report. It would not work. I tried various ways, but the only thing to do was to take it into the cabin for drying out and testing. I unscrewed it and carried it aft. At that moment I suddenly began to feel sea-sick. I handed the radio to Ross and lay down, feeling fit again at once. Ross played with its innards and inserted a new valve, but after sitting up he, too, suddenly felt ill. All of us were fit when lying down, but each felt seedy the moment he sat up and tried to do anything.

A second episode took place during a race across the Bay of Biscay, a notoriously "retched" body of water.

> We started on a brilliant Sunday afternoon with a fine fresh breeze to shake us down. The wind headed in the early hours of Monday morning and by 0830 it had freshened so much that we had to take in a reef. We kept the genoa standing, but the bolt holding the runner plate sheared under the strain and repairs had to be effected. At 1000 the mainsail tore right across under the headboard. The sail came down with a run and the headboard and halyard went aloft to the masthead.
>
> *Cohoe*'s mast was solid, high and thin, and above the jumpers it was little more than the thickness of a big walking stick. A considerable swell was running and a fairly rough sea, so there was no prospect of swarming up the mast to retrieve the halyard. The burgee sheave was a strong one, so we tried to lead a wire rope through it by means of the burgee halyard, but the attempts were unsuccessful and finally the burgee halyard broke.
>
> We then shackled the bosun's chair to the fore halyard and hoisted Dick Trafford, the lightest of the three of us, up to the forestay block. But the motion was so wild aloft and he was thrown about so much that he could not reach the peak and retrieve the main halyard. When he was lowered to the deck he was violently sick.
>
> Deprived of her mainsail, the yacht was rolling tremendously in the seas. It was difficult to retain one's foothold even on deck, and aloft, even when secured to the mast, it was like being at the end of a pendulum, as it swung first one side and then the other over the sea. It was enough to make anybody sea-sick.
>
> We abandoned the attempts to retrieve the main halyard and lashed the mainsail to the boom. Next we tried setting the trysail by means of the spinnaker halyard, but this failed because we could not get the lead right.

Only one thing was left that could be done and that was to reeve a new halyard through a block and lash the block to the mast above the upper spreader. When the block and halyard were ready Ross volunteered to go aloft with them, but Dick and I did not relish the idea of pulling over 13 stone in weight up the mast by means of the fore halyard; nor would it have been fair on the small mast winch. Accordingly, I, as the next lightest, went up in the bosun's chair. This was quickly done with the aid of Ross's and Dick's beef at the winch. Like Dick, I found the motion aloft made things difficult. I really needed both hands to hold on by, but I got a temporary grip with my knees round the mast when lashing the block in position. The repair was a strong one and I was soon on deck again, when I, too, was promptly sick. All three of us had now been sick, which after all was a compliment to the tremendous parties we had enjoyed in Spain.[3]

Both accounts support the sensory conflict theory of seasickness. No other theory can explain the occurrence of seasickness after awakening and feeling "well and refreshed." This phenomenon is not uncommon. Seasickness may first rear its ugly head after the sailor awakes. Or the sailor may lie down *because* of seasickness and awake feeling much better, only to have the symptoms recur as soon as he gets up. This postsleep seasickness would certainly rule out a psychological cause!

The second account is convincing evidence against the overstimulation theory. Vestibular stimulation surely must be greater while swinging like a pendulum from the top of the mast than down on deck. Why then did the seasickness occur in at least two of the three sailors only when they had returned to the deck? Most likely, the pendulumlike swinging was somewhat independent of the motion of the boat and did not produce enough sensory conflict, whereas the re-exposure to the abnormal boat movements (after an absence) was sufficient. The parties in Spain undoubtedly had nothing to do with the seasickness.

These two episodes also highlight the difficulty of predicting when seasickness will occur in those of us who are generally immune (and Coles would seem to be in the "hardly ever" category). After all, the people at each end of the spectrum present no challenge. Some fortunate individuals have yet to experience their own Waterloo—although if their vestibular systems are intact, there is no reason to suppose that they are *totally* immune. At the opposite end of the spectrum are those people who are extremely susceptible. They tend to be weeded out early and avoid water travel at all costs—which was not an easy proposition just 50 years ago!

Most sailors fall between these extremes. It would be helpful if we could identify the particular factors that induce seasickness in each person. Possibly some people are more susceptible to the vestibular, visual, and neck-position conflict, whereas others possess less tolerance for the canal-U&S conflict. So far, however, this is merely speculation. Until studies are made, all we can do is to try to eliminate *each* of the known precipitating factors.

The effect of the size of the vessel on seasickness has received little experimentation. Nevertheless, it is well known that some people tend to be more susceptible to seasickness on either small or large boats. In fact, the sensory rearrangement that occurs in the motion analyzer is quite specific. For example, adaptation to the motion of an ocean liner by no means guarantees protection in a 100-foot yacht or small sailboat (and vice versa). Each situation presents the motion analyzer with a new learning experience.

In any given sea, individual variation determines who becomes sick, as well as the severity and duration of the symptoms. We can make a few generalizations, however. Women tend to be more susceptible than men to all forms of motion sickness, including seasickness. Women are at even higher risk during menstruation and pregnancy, suggesting that hormonal changes play some, as yet unexplained, role. There are also age-related differences in susceptibility. Children below the age of 2 are almost totally immune. The risk then increases throughout childhood until adolescence, when it begins to decline *slowly*. The elderly are fairly immune.

Regardless of these general trends, we are all aware that there is much individual variation, which depends on two factors: susceptibility and adaptation. If the motion is weak (a mild sea swell), the most susceptible are usually the first to develop head symptoms (such as skin pallor, cold sweating, and dizziness), which may be followed by gut symptoms. Resistant crew members may develop only head symptoms or nothing at all. With a severe stimulus (for example, when a boat leaves a protected harbor and heads directly into a rough sea), the more sensitive people tend to develop nausea and vomiting right away. The head symptoms may be overshadowed completely.

The ability to adapt, as well as the rapidity with which adaptation takes place, is an individual trait. The motion analyzer is usually able to reconcile the chaos within about 72 hours, but a minority remains seasick for an entire journey. Fortunately, this occurs in less than 5 percent of the population.

In general, people exhibit these traits in four varying combinations: (1) high susceptibility/fast adaptation, which yields an initially severe reaction that diminishes rapidly; (2) high susceptibility/slow adaptation, the worst combination! (3) low susceptibility/slow adaptation, which produces prolonged head symptoms sometimes intermittently punctuated by nausea and vomiting; and (4) low susceptibility/fast adaptation, the ideal combination.

ON THE WRONG TACK

Since motion sickness is due to sensory conflict, a number of myths can now be jettisoned. Because the stomach is an "innocent bystander," dietary prescriptions and proscriptions are not necessary. In the past, a wide variety of absurd diets was prescribed for the embarking passenger. These varied between gastronomic austerity—dry toast or gruel—and gastronomic whimsy—"soup made of horse radish and rice, seasoned with red herrings and sardines."[4] The latter was to be washed down with a "light, sparkling wine."

There is no evidence that diet has any effect on seasickness whatsoever. To this we may add two codicils however. Any drugs, foods, or odors that by themselves can cause either nausea or disequilibrium, including alcohol, should be avoided. Also, it has been suggested that an empty stomach may slightly increase the risk of seasickness. Scientific evidence is not conclusive on this point, and it may not make any difference. It certainly doesn't matter *what* is put into the stomach, despite the fact that some people swear by certain foods, such as dry crackers or flat cola drink.[5]

A popular belief is that cold weather predisposes to seasickness. However, ambient temperature (both warm and cold) has not been found to influence susceptibility.

It has been suggested that removal of wax from the external ear canal is beneficial. Although extensive ear wax might impair hearing, there is no reason why it should have any effect on balance. The inner ear is tucked away inside the skull and is not normally in direct contact with the ear canal.

One particularly dangerous and nonsensical form of treatment is the patching of one eye. It may be derived from the sensory conflict theory. Perhaps someone thought that there would be less conflict if there were only half as much vision (not true). In any case, forget it.

Another voodoo therapy that is on the market is the so-called seasick strap, a device worn on each wrist. "Acupressure" is applied to the anatomical points on the wrist that purportedly diminish nausea. Like most of these forms of therapy, claims are made, but adequate studies, with control groups including a placebo, are not available.

One particularly widespread misconception is that emotional stress and anxiety predispose to seasickness. This belief has several origins. First, there is a group of people who have *psychological* motion sickness. These individuals become nauseated and may vomit at the sight (or even the thought!) of a boat. Such symptoms indicate a form of neurosis, however, and not true motion sickness. One writer has suggested the term *emotion sickness* for the illness these people suffer. Second, fear or anxiety is a handy explanation, despite the fact that it is usually wrong. Most combat troops in World War II, for example, erroneously attributed their motion sickness to fear, even though they readily admitted that they did not remember feeling particularly fearful at the time. The third origin is cultural. At least since the 19th century, seasickness has been regarded as evidence of a "lack of moral fiber," or worse yet, a failure of "intestinal fortitude." This is evident from a few lines of the *HMS Pinafore* libretto:

> Though related to a peer
> I can hand, reef, and steer
> And ship a selvagee
> I am never known to quail
> At the fury of a gale
> And I'm never, never sick at sea![6]

The stigma of unmanliness continues to pervade our attitude toward the seasick individual. Although it is true that anxiety may worsen the situation, *the basic mechanism of seasickness is not psychological.* History certainly bears this out. Only 4 years before the Battle of Trafalgar, Lord Nelson (no shrinking violet) wrote, "Heavy sea, sick to death—this sea sickness I shall never get over." It is safe to say that he never did, since he was even seasick on the voyage to his final battle at Trafalgar!

TREATMENT

Cicero once opined that he "would rather be killed than suffer the tortures of *nausea maris.*" This statement may seem rather draconian to those of you who have never been sick, but anyone who has suffered a severe and prolonged attack can identify with the sentiment. The recurring theme is one of hopelessness, despair, and a yearning for an end to it all. It is easy to imagine how this attitude could adversely affect survival.

Preventive Medicine

We cannot completely prevent seasickness. If the sea conditions are violent enough, almost everyone will succumb. However, before rushing headlong into drug treatment, there are some simple precautions that should be con-

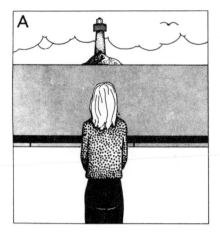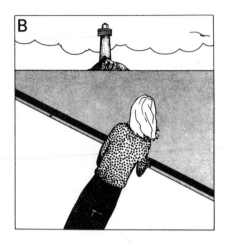

Figure 1.7. Rolling motion to starboard without visual-vestibular conflict.

sidered. If you are responsible for the safety of the boat and crew, it may be worthwhile to question the crew, prior to departure, about previous episodes of seasickness. If they have had no previous sea exposure, the presence or absence of car sickness or of other forms of motion sickness can serve as a rough guide. As a rule, if the crew member is able to read in a moving car, he is probably not overly susceptible. Conversely, susceptibility to car sickness indicates a propensity toward seasickness.

In a similar vein, it is prudent to anticipate the sea conditions that will be encountered en route. For example, if the temperature is expected to fall or heavy weather is anticipated, crew members should be advised to err on the side of overdressing. It is far easier to shed excessive clothing and hand it below during rough conditions than it is to go below and change, especially to the forward cabin.

As we have seen, anxiety does not cause seasickness—but it can exacerbate it. One experiment demonstrated that the incidence of seasickness is lower in subjects who were given a task to perform than in subjects who were not. In another experiment, subjects who were encouraged to pay attention to the abnormal motions were invariably sick. Thus, when feasible, crew members should be kept busy. It is no time for rumination!

Any maneuver that diminishes sensory conflict may ameliorate the seasickness. For this reason, staying on deck should be encouraged, and not simply to get fresh air as most people suppose. If during a rolling motion to starboard, for example, vision is directed at a stationary point on land or at the horizon, sensory conflict does not occur (Figure 1.7). Both the vestibular system and the visual system register the same rolling motion. It is of no value to look at the mast or any other part of the boat. The object must be stationary with respect to the earth.

Thus seasickness is frequently lessened by taking the helm. The helmsman has a task that distracts him from his sickness and at the same time requires him to keep an eye on the horizon. This active role lessens the chance for seasickness and may even ameliorate the condition once it is present. Experimental evidence corroborates the fact that sensory rearrangement is facilitated by active participation. It is true of all forms of motion sickness that the operator of the vehicle (in this case, the boat) is less apt to become sick than are the passengers.

Parenthetically, car sickness in children is probably also due to sensory conflict. Since a child is often unable to see out of the front window, particularly from the back seat, he or she experiences an analogous vestibular-visual conflict. A car seat, which elevates the child, can alleviate the problem.

If being below deck during turbulence cannot be avoided, it is advisable to keep the eyes closed to eliminate some of the conflict. If head movements are restrained, the conflict is lessened further. Several studies have now shown that restricting head movements eliminates signals from the third source of information—the neck position sensors. More important, it reduces the semicircular canal–U&S conflict to a great degree. Simply holding the head against the back of a seat, if high enough, is often sufficient neck restriction.

If things continue to go from bad to worse, the best advice is to lie down, face up, eyes closed, as close to the middle of the boat as possible. This position will diminish most of the conflict, including some—but by no means all—of the intrinsic canal–U&S conflict as well. Lying down, however, slows down the natural adaptation response. As we have seen, the adaptation response functions more rapidly as an *active* rather than a *passive* process. Therefore, if the crew member can "tough it out," preferably by keeping busy, he will be better off in the long run.[7]

Drug Treatment

Modern drug treatment for seasickness had an unexpected inception. In 1947 a woman was being treated for hives with the antihistamine dimenhydrinate (Dramamine). She noticed that she was serendipitously cured of her car sickness every time she took the drug! Her physicians reported this phenomenon, and the next year was to witness "Operation Nausea," a full-scale trial of Dramamine conducted on a troopship crossing the Atlantic during a storm. So began modern drug therapy for seasickness.

Although there is no single, ideal anti-motion-sickness drug, a number are very effective (Table 1.2). Of course, individuals vary in their response to each of these drugs; thus, the only way to determine the drug or drugs and the dosage that are best for any individual is by trial and error. In order to make an intelligent choice, these concepts should be kept in mind:

1. The goal is to maximize the anti-motion-sickness properties of a drug and to minimize its side effects. Because of a high recommended dosage, scopolamine, the oldest and still the most effective anti-motion-sickness medication, has received unwarranted "bad press" for many years. Previously, the recommended dosage was about twice as high as is actually necessary, and nearly everyone experienced significant side effects as a result!

2. None of these drugs acts immediately. It takes time for the drug to *begin* to act, and even longer for it to provide *maximal* protection. For example, Dramamine requires at least 2 hours before there is any anti-motion-sickness effect. In a short-term situation, it would be illogical to expect Dramamine to be of any use. However, scopolamine, which is effective rapidly, would be an intelligent choice.

3. A corollary to number 2 is that different drugs have different durations of action. Dramamine offers longer protection than scopolamine. For most of these drugs, the duration of action is inversely related to the time it takes for the drug to act. Obviously, a drug with a short duration of action has to be repeated at more frequent intervals than a drug with a long duration of action.

The most effective preparation tested so far is the combination of 0.3 to 0.6 milligram scopolamine plus 5 to 10 milligrams dextroamphetamine. This combination has in fact been prescribed for astronauts suffering from space sickness. It has been thoroughly tested in seasickness, and, for susceptible people under rough conditions, this is the treatment of choice.

There are, however, some minor problems with the combination. The duration of action is only about 4 hours (which means that repeated doses are necessary), and it is becoming difficult to obtain dextroamphetamine because of its potential for drug abuse. The side effects of scopolamine include drowsiness, blurred vision, and dry mouth (and, rarely, dizziness, rapid heart rate, urinary obstruction, and worsening of glaucoma). But the side effects are usually a problem only with high doses or in very young or old people. Initially the dextroamphetamine was added simply to

TABLE 1.2
Anti-Motion-Sickness Drugs*

Drugs	Dosage (mg)	Duration of Action (hrs)	Indications
Dramamine	50	6	Mild sensitivity and/or sea conditions.
Marezine	50	6	Pretreatment necessary. Doses approximately 8 hrs and 2 hrs before departure may be optimal.
Meclizine	25–50	6–12	
Phenergan** and Ephedrine	25 25	6–12	Moderate sensitivity and/or sea conditions.
Scopolamine** and Dextroamphetamine**	0.3–0.6 5–10	4	Severe sensitivity and/or sea conditions.
Phenergan Suppository	25	6–12	Probably the treatment of choice when nausea and vomiting are already present.
Transderm-Scopolamine	0.5	72	Mainly for prophylaxis. Should be applied the night prior to departure.

*See Appendix for common drug equivalents.
**Also effective when used alone.

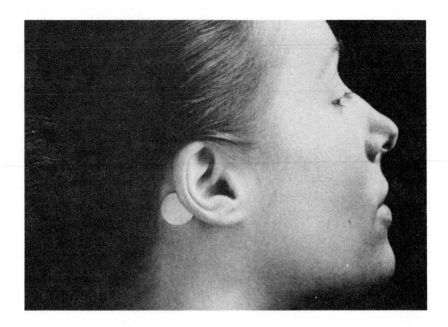

Figure 1.8. Transderm-scopolamine disk in place. (*Courtesy of CIBA-GEIGY*)

counteract the drowsiness the scopolamine produced, but recent experiments have demonstrated that dextroamphetamine has significant anti-motion-sickness properties of its own. In fact, it is second in effectiveness only to scopolamine. The important side effects of dextroamphetamine are insomnia and hyperactivity (sometimes with insufferable loquaciousness!). The scopolamine tends to counteract and modify both of these symptoms.

Only slightly less effective is the combination of 25 milligrams promethazine (Phenergan) plus 25 milligrams ephedrine. The duration of action is approximately twice as long, which is a definite advantage. The side effects are similar, but not as marked. Phenergan alone may produce drowsiness, and ephedrine may produce a slight "high," although not nearly as much as dextroamphetamine. As in the first combination, these drugs were chosen to counteract each other's side effects. This combination is becoming very popular throughout the nautical community.

Three of the above drugs—scopolamine, dextroamphetamine, and Phenergan—have proven effectiveness by themselves. Scopolamine and Phenergan can be given intramuscularly, and Phenergan is available as a suppository, a very effective route of administration.

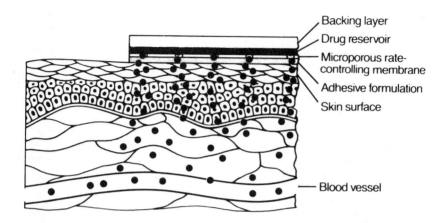

Backing layer
Drug reservoir
Microporous rate-controlling membrane
Adhesive formulation
Skin surface
Blood vessel

Figure 1.9. Cross section of skin surface with schematic illustration of the transdermal scopolamine system. (Courtesy of CIBA-GEIGY)

Scientists have recently developed a new method for administering scopolamine. An adhesive, transdermal disk containing the drug is applied to a hairless spot on the skin, usually behind the ear for convenience (Figure 1.8). The drug is slowly absorbed through the skin into the bloodstream (Figure 1.9). The idea behind the transdermal system is that a low-dose, continuous administration maintains an effective level in the bloodstream while it reduces the side effects. The system delivers 0.5 milligram over a period of 3 days. Since it generally takes 2 to 4 hours after application to achieve an effective concentration, the disk must be applied at least that long before exposure. CIBA-GEIGY, the manufacturer, recommends applying the disk up to 12 hours before, or the night prior to, departure. The disk is impervious to water and may be worn while swimming or showering. Once removed, however, it cannot be reused. The side effects do seem to be less, but they are still present. Dry mouth in two out of three cases and drowsiness in about one out of six cases are quite usual. Blurred vision is also common.

There are three antihistamines (available without a prescription) that are about equally effective when used in mild to moderate situations: (1) dimenhydrinate (Dramamine)—50 milligrams; (2) cyclizine (Marezine)—50 milligrams; and (3) meclizine (Bonine, Antivert)—25 to 50 milligrams. It is recommended that they be administered at least 2 hours before exposure, but there is evidence that pretreatment the day before may be even better.

We still do not know precisely how these drugs prevent or at least ameliorate seasickness. It is clear that they alter the sensitivity of the central nervous system rather than of either the semicircular canals or the U&S, as was once supposed. Functionally, these drugs "pacify" the motion analyzer, allowing the sailor to experience the abnormal motion for a longer period of time without becoming sick. This means that the brain has more time to adapt to the motion—and *adaptation is the only cure.*

If you are preparing a first-aid kit, it is important to include at least one drug that can be taken nonorally. Unless a physician or nurse is available, intramuscular injections are not feasible. Phenergan suppositories are a rapid, effective, and practical alternative. So is the transdermal scopolamine system, although it is at least 2 hours before a significant amount of the drug is absorbed.

Except for the antihistamines, all of the seasickness drugs discussed earlier require a prescription. At the recommended dosages, these drugs are fairly safe for young, healthy adults. For very young children, older adults, or anyone with medical problems, the choice should be made in concert with a physician.

CODA

During a severe episode of seasickness, the feeling of hopelessness and despair can be overwhelming. If you should find yourself in such a state, you need only consider the fate of a young Englishman who became violently seasick during his first ocean voyage. In a letter to his father, a physician, the youth wrote:

We sailed, as you know, on the 27th of December, and have been fortunate enough to have had from that time to the present a fair and moderate breeze. It afterwards proved that we had escaped a heavy gale in the Channel, another at Madeira, and another on the Coast of Africa. But in escaping the gale, we felt its consequence—a heavy sea. In the Bay of Biscay there was a long and continuous swell, and the misery I endured from sea-sickness is far beyond what I ever guessed at. I believe you are curious about it. I will give you all my dear-bought experience. Nobody who has only been to sea for twenty-four hours has a right to say that sea-sickness is even uncomfortable. The real misery only begins when you are so exhausted that a little exertion makes a feeling of faintness come on. I found nothing but lying in my hammock did me any good.

...In short, I find a ship a very comfortable house, with everything you want, and if it was not for sea-sickness the whole world would be sailors. I do not think there is much danger of Erasmus setting the example, but in case there should be, he may rely upon it he does not know one-tenth of the sufferings of sea-sickness.

[Letter from Charles Darwin to his father, dated February 8, 1832, written aboard the HMS *Beagle*][8]

NOTES

1. The following note is for biology aficionados (others may safely skip). The most instructive and widely used paradigm for motion sickness is the *Coriolis vestibular reaction*. The Coriolis reaction is produced by simultaneous rotation about two perpendicular axes. If the term sounds vaguely familiar, it should, since the Coriolis force is in good part responsible for our weather patterns. Because of angular rotation of the earth, northerly or southerly air masses are deflected to the right in the Northern Hemisphere and to the left in the Southern Hemisphere. The Coriolis vestibular reaction is similar. As we have seen, horizontal rotation to the left, as in a rotating chair, initially stimulates the left horizontal canal and inhibits the right. However, if rotation is continued at constant velocity (zero acceleration), the endolymph will eventually overcome its inertia and acquire the same velocity as the canal itself. At this point the cupula will spring back to its neutral position. If, during this constant velocity rotation to the left, the person tilts his head to the right shoulder, a seemingly bizarre phenomenon occurs— motion sickness! Actually, most people need more than one tilt to become sick.

The explanation lies in the incompatibility of the information the canals and U&S supply. When the head is tilted to the right shoulder, the U&S, unaffected by the rotation, signal right head tilt. All well and good. But with the head tilted, we now bring the two anterior canals into the plane of rotation and they are stimulated. But stimulation of the anterior canals usually occurs when the head is rotated forward. There's the rub. The U&S are signaling head tilt to the right while the canals are signaling forward head rotation. The only way this could occur is if the head were split down the middle and each half flew off in different directions! No wonder the brain becomes perplexed.

It might be asked how this is comparable to our experience on the water, since even in the roughest weather we are never subjected to this kind of stimulus. True, the assault on our vestibular system is not as regular or predictable; however, the same kind of semicircular canal and U&S "conflict" occurs on a smaller scale over a much longer period of time. The Coriolis vestibular reaction can produce nausea and vomiting in less than a minute, whereas seasickness usually takes about 30 minutes or more to occur.

2. For a recent comprehensive review of the subject, see J. T. Reason and J. J. Brand, *Motion Sickness* (New York: Academic Press, 1975). Professor Reason has also published a text intended for a general readership, *Man in Motion: The Psychology of Travel* (New York: Walker, 1974), and a technical review entitled "Motion Sickness Adaptation: A Neural Mismatch Model," in *Journal of the Royal Society of Medicine* 71 (1978):819-829.

3. K. A. Coles, *Heavy Weather Sailing,* 3d rev. ed., 1981 (Clinton Corners, N.Y.: De Graff, and London: Adlard Coles, Ltd.), pp. 73-74, 82-83.

4. J. T. Reason and J. J. Brand, *Motion Sickness* (New York: Academic Press, 1975), p. 10.

5. The latest proposed cure for motion sickness is powdered ginger root, see D. B. Mowrey and D. E. Clayson, "Motion sickness, ginger, and psycho-physics," *Lancet* 1 (1982):655-657. The authors suggest that "ginger ameliorates the effects of motion sickness in the gastrointestinal tract itself. It may increase gastric motility and absorb neutralizing toxins and acids, so effectively blocking gastrointestinal reactions and subsequent nausea feedback." Unless that makes more sense to you

than it does to me, I would refrain from stocking up on ginger root at the present time.

6. *The Complete Plays of Gilbert and Sullivan* (New York: Garden City, 1938), p. 105.

7. In two other motion sickness situations (aircraft pilot sickness and spacecraft sickness), adaptation schedules have been developed. These individuals are gradually exposed in the laboratory to increasing stimuli of the sort that they are likely to encounter in the air or in space. In these two situations, the types of abnormal motion are limited and stereotyped, and adaptation exposures do confer some protection. Since the abnormal motion that occurs on the water is anything but stereotyped, adaptation schedules for sailors have not been very helpful. Perhaps sailors can hasten the adaptation response somewhat by sleeping aboard the night prior to departure. Yet it is doubtful whether this will offer much protection against really heavy weather.

8. F. Darwin (Ed.), *The Autobiography of Charles Darwin and Selected Letters* (New York: Dover, 1958), pp. 135-137.

2

Cold Weather Sailing

The sea lies all around us.... In its myster-
ious past it encompasses all the dim origins
of life and receives in the end, after, it may
be, many transmutations, the dead husks of
that same life. For all at last returns to the
sea—the beginning and the end.

Rachel Carson, *The Sea Around Us,* 1951

CONSIDER THE SINKING OF the *Titanic* in 1912. The water temperature was approximately 32° F (0° C) when the ship foundered. When rescue vessels arrived 2 hours later, nearly all of the people who entered lifeboats were alive. In contrast, all of the 1,489 people immersed in the water appeared to be (and were presumed to be) dead. We now know that the victims suffered from hypothermia and that many could probably have been revived! Insufficient clothing, a lack of adequate flotation devices, and an absence of even a rudimentary knowledge of cold-water-survival procedures all contributed to the high death toll.

As sailors we must learn to deal with the cold in two different circumstances. *On the water* while sailing, a foolhardy approach to the cold decreases comfort and impairs performance. Although our lives are not directly in peril, impaired performance certainly may have untoward consequences. *In the water,* we are engaged in a battle for survival. In either case, we have no excuse for not knowing how to keep ourselves warm.

THERMAL BALANCE ON THE WATER

Man is a homoiothermic, or warm-blooded, animal whose internal temperature is normally kept within narrow limits despite the vagaries of the climate. This he accomplishes by balancing heat gain with heat loss. When successful, man is in thermal balance with his environment.[1]

In a cold environment, the human body is in danger of losing heat faster than it can be produced. Unless something is done, the body continues to cool off until a state of *hypothermia* supervenes. In order to decide upon appropriate measures to arrest this loss of body heat, let us consider the ways in which the body gains and loses heat (Table 2.1).

The most obvious source of heat is *metabolism.* An average adult man produces about 3,000 calories of energy per day performing various light activities such as sleeping, eating, dressing, and walking. About 95 percent of this energy is in the form of heat. Exposure to the cold does not affect the basic rate of metabolism very much. After weeks or months in the cold, the rate of metabolism may increase a small amount, but this increase does not provide protection against hypothermia. Interestingly, a few groups in the world have been able to adapt, with almost no protection, to extremely frigid conditions by increasing their metabolism, although the evidence for this is scanty. One such group, the natives of Tierra del Fuego (Cape Horn), live in an intensely cold, windy, and wet climate. The temperature is near freezing the entire year. Darwin visited them during his voyage on the H.M.S. *Beagle,* noting that the Fuegian men and women were almost completely naked. "A woman, who was suckling a recently-born child, came one day alongside the vessel, and remained there out of mere curiosity, whilst the sleet fell and thawed on her naked bosom and on the skin of her naked baby!"[2] Their higher rate of metabolism allows the Fuegians to survive in this thoroughly unpleasant climate.

A second means of increasing heat production is muscular activity— either *shivering* or *exercise.* Shivering is involuntary and begins soon after exposure to the cold. It reaches a peak in about 15 to 30 minutes and increases heat production 2 to 3 times. Vigorous exercise is more efficient. It may increase heat production 10 times. Shivering and exercise are not additive, however, since exercise usually abolishes shivering.

TABLE 2.1
Heat Gain and Heat Loss

Heat Gain	Heat Loss
Metabolism	Radiation
Shivering or Exercise	Convection
Radiation	Conduction
Ingestion of Hot Food	Evaporation

There are two other means by which the body can gain heat—by the absorption of heat *radiation* and by the consumption of *hot food and beverages.* During the daytime the body receives shortwave radiation from the sun, both direct and reflected. It also may absorb longwave radiation.

Finally, eating hot food and drinking hot beverages supply heat to the body. In *Two Years Before the Mast,* R. H. Dana describes that in a cold environment sailors invariably prefer a hot beverage to an alcoholic one. "At the same time, as I have said, there was not a man on board who would not have pitched the rum to the dogs (I have heard them say so a dozen times) for a pot of coffee or chocolate; or even for our common beverage—'water bewitched and tea begrudged,' as it was."[3]

Conversely, there are four ways in which the body loses heat: radiation, convection, conduction, and evaporation—all of which are important on the water (Figure 2.1). Regardless of skin color, the human body not only absorbs but emits longwave *radiation.* This exchange is not generally appreciated. When the surface of the body is not absorbing longwave radiation, it is actually radiating it back into the environment. The degree of radiation heat loss depends on the amount of exposed body surface, which is usually 80 percent or less, since certain areas such as the thighs and underarms tend to radiate heat back to the body. Curling up in a fetal position diminishes radiation heat loss. Lying spread-eagled enhances it.

Convection is the other important means by which the sailor loses heat. Air that is in direct contact with the skin is warmed. As it is warmed it rises off the skin surface and is replaced by cooler air. These convection currents maintain themselves by transferring heat from the skin to the surrounding air. The amount of heat loss depends on the temperature difference between the skin and the air; the larger the difference, the greater the heat loss. Wind velocity also plays a role. Although convection currents occur even when there is no wind whatsoever (e.g., in a telephone

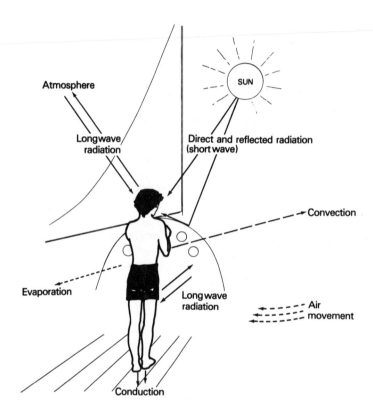

Figure 2.1. The four avenues of heat loss: radiation, convection, conduction, and evaporation.

booth), increasing the movement of air across the skin hastens the exchange of heat. Birds and some mammals are able to decrease convection heat loss to an enormous extent by fluffing up their feathers or bristling their hair. The goose-bumps phenomenon we experience in the cold is a vestige of this response, although, unfortunately, it adds nothing to our insulation.

Conduction heat loss occurs when the body is in direct contact with a cooler object. Heat is transferred directly to the object. On the water, conduction is usually insignificant, since only the sailor's feet and/or buttocks are in contact with a cooler object, such as the boat. In the water, the situation is drastically different. Now, nearly the entire body is in contact with the colder water, and conduction becomes the most important avenue for heat loss.

Evaporation plays a vital role in cooling the body in a warm climate, but it is of lesser consequence in the cold. In cold climates, sweating usually does not occur, although water vapor continually diffuses through the skin without wetting it. This evaporation, together with water vapor emitted from the respiratory tract, is known as insensible water loss because we are entirely unaware of it. Since the evaporation of water requires heat, this heat is lost from the body. In the cold, this evaporative heat loss generally is minimal. However, there are circumstances (discussed later in this chapter) when it may be a major source of heat loss.

NATURAL DEFENSES AGAINST THE COLD

It is useful to think of the human body as a warm central "core" surrounded by a cooler "shell" (Figure 2.2). The core contains all of the vital organs, whereas the shell consists of the skin, underlying subcutaneous tissues, and muscles. The shell provides the body with a layer of natural insulation, which *varies to suit the climate*. In warm climates the shell is very thin so that heat from the core quickly dissipates. In cold weather the core "retreats" to a more defensible position in the interior, leaving behind a thick shell to fight a rearguard action with the elements. The flow of blood controls the size of the shell, which can change very rapidly and constitutes our first response to cold and hot temperatures. Warm blood from the core may be directed toward or diverted away from the surface. When diverted away, the insulation of the outer inch of the body—the shell—approaches that of cork! Since the blood brings less heat to the surface, the temperature of the skin falls and less heat is lost.

Sailors should be aware that *alcohol decreases the size of the shell and should be avoided in the cold*. It does this by dilating blood vessels, hence

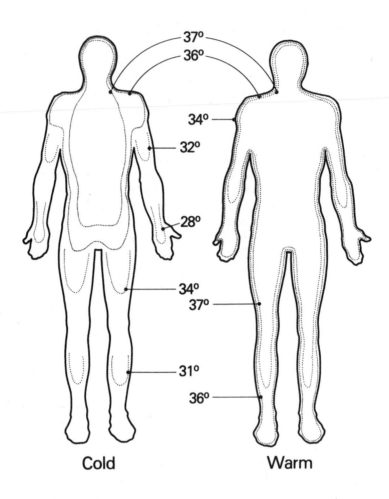

Figure 2.2. The distribution of the shell and the core in cold and warm weather. (Measurements are in degrees Centigrade.)

increasing blood flow to the skin—precisely what the body is trying to avoid! An account of a vessel's sinking in the North Atlantic during the month of October demonstrates the detrimental effect of alcohol. "There were forty of us on or clinging to a fifteen-man Carley float. Rescue came after seven hours. There was only one casualty, an able seaman who had drunk rum just before abandoning ship. He died after about three hours' immersion."[4]

If increasing the size of the shell fails to stem the tide, the body turns to its second line of defense, increased heat production either by shivering or exercise. Exercise is a potent resource, increasing heat production up to 10 times; however, problems can arise. First, exercise tolerance varies markedly among individuals depending on their physical fitness. Some people may be able to sustain vigorous activity for long periods of time (keeping themselves warm in the process), whereas others simply become exhausted. The second drawback is that some of the heat is wasted. During physical activity, blood must be supplied to the muscles, diminishing the insulation of the shell and nullifying some of the heat gain. As a general rule, if the heat loss is modest, exercise may produce enough of a net gain in heat to keep the sailor warm. If the heat loss is proceeding at a rapid pace, chances are that exercise will be counterproductive. One situation in which exercise is nearly always counterproductive is during immersion in cool or cold water.

IMMERSION HYPOTHERMIA

Most sailors never stop to consider hypothermia unless they are sailing in high-latitude waters in the wintertime. This is a mistake. *Even when sailing in tropical waters, hypothermia remains a potential hazard.* Figure 2.3 represents the change in body temperature of a thin man swimming in water of various temperatures. Note that his body temperature drops precipitously in cold water, but that even in water temperatures as high as 83° F (28° C) the swimmer continues to lose heat, albeit very slowly. Figure 2.4 is a widely used diagram for estimating the survival time for a fully clothed, average-sized man in cold water. The two important variables are the temperature of the water and the duration of immersion. Thin men have shorter survival times, whereas fatter men and most women have slightly longer times due to the additional insulation of extra adipose tissue. Improving the type and amount of clothing and wearing a waterproof outer suit further increase survival time.

The following incident illustrates how a misunderstanding of some of

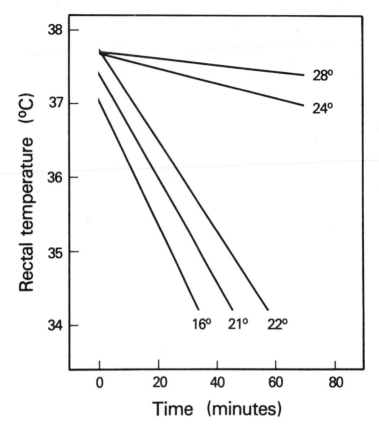

Figure 2.3. Body heat loss for a thin, unclothed swimmer at various water temperatures. In colder water (16° C, 21° C, 22° C), heat loss proceeds at a rapid rate; in warmer water (24° C, 28° C), at a slow rate.

the concepts of cold water survival can be tragic. Adlard Coles documents it in *Heavy Weather Sailing.* A vessel, the *Dancing Ledge,* foundered during a midsummer gale in the English Channel. An experienced sailor, Lieutenant-Colonel H. Barry O'Sullivan, his wife, and two crew members were sailing her. The vessel broke up very rapidly, leaving little time for preparation. Mrs. O'Sullivan recounts:

> Once in the fresh air, we saw each other fairly soon, and also saw the dinghy, which must have broken from its chocks on the cabin top. It was upside down, but we hung on to it (aided by life-jackets) for nearly four hours and were carried inshore until we were close enough to see the window panes

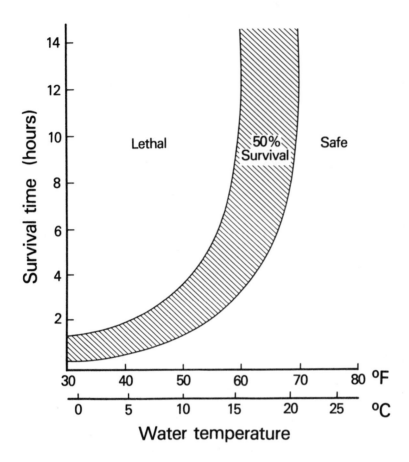

Figure 2.4. *Predicted survival in cold water. The two most important considerations are: (1) time in the water and (2) water temperature. To use this graph, draw a line for a specific water temperature vertically until it intersects either curve. A horizontal line indicates the probable survival time. For example, if the water temperature is 55° F (13° C), there is a 50 percent chance for survival at 2 hours. By 6 hours the chance for survival approaches 0.*

on the Ventnor houses....Barry insisted that we should "bicycle" continuously with our legs to keep warm and avoid stomach cramp, which it proved successful in doing.

According to Coles:

The youngest member of the crew had only a kapok life-jacket. This proved to be totally inadequate and as he became cold and weak his head had no support. Colonel and Mrs. O'Sullivan held on to the dinghy with one hand, and supported the crew's head with the other. The fourth member of the crew had already died.

A frigate, H.M.S. *Keppel*, approached at about this time. Colonel .O'Sullivan took off his orange jacket to wave it above the spray to attract attention and this was seen as a tiny dot by the naval watch. He then attempted to put it onto the exhausted member of the crew to give him chin support, and he had therefore no jacket for himself.

When the frigate was manoeuvred alongside (no mean feat), a rope was thrown to Mrs. O'Sullivan. She let go the dinghy with one hand to grip the rope. Her hand was so cold and rigid that she could not close it round the rope. She let go the dinghy with the other hand to attempt to get a stronger grip, but it was impossible to hold the rope and it ran through her hands as a wave, deflected by the bulk of the frigate, swept her along the length of the ship and she drifted away into the clear, supported by her life-jacket, and became unconscious. The frigate returned and Mrs. O'Sullivan was rescued by a man, secured by a lifeline, who went into the water and got her up the scrambling nets. The search was continued for the others, but there was no trace of the dinghy or the men.[5]

What should the sailor do when faced with the necessity of entering cold water? The foundering of the *Dancing Ledge* was exceptional in that the vessel broke up so rapidly. Usually there are at least a few minutes for preparation, during which time as much warm clothing as possible should be donned, including a cap and a waterproof outer suit if available.[6] A personal flotation device (PFD) is mandatory. It will help the sailor retain the energy—and thus the heat—to stay afloat. If he should become unconscious, it will keep his head out of the water and prevent drowning. For want of a life jacket, the captain of the *Dancing Ledge* lost his life.

Next, if the water temperature is below 50° F (10° C), gloves and shoes should be worn. These are required because of a curious phenomenon known as cold vasodilatation. As we have seen, diverting blood from the shell to the core reduces heat loss. This diversion is caused by the constriction of the blood vessels of the skin (vasoconstriction). However, when the cold is severe enough to damage the hands and feet, vasoconstriction periodically gives way to vasodilatation (about every 20 minutes). Presumably this periodic "rewarming" of the fingers and toes developed to protect these exposed and vulnerable appendages. Unfortunately, in the process of saving the fingers and toes, a tremendous amount of heat is lost; thus the need for gloves and shoes.

If there is time, it is worthwhile to take a rapidly acting seasickness preparation, since seasickness promotes heat loss.

Rather than jump in, the sailor should lower himself gradually if possible. Occasionally, strong, physically fit individuals have died almost immediately after entering very cold water. The cause is unknown, but some of the deaths seem to be due to a reflex hyperventilation (overbreathing) produced by intense cold. These individuals experience difficulty breathing, suddenly flounder in the water, and drown.

As soon as the sailor enters the water, his body loses heat at a much more rapid rate. Since his head remains out of the water, it continues to lose heat at about the same rate as before immersion (primarily by radiation and convection). In the water, the body also loses some heat via radiation and convection, but now conduction plays the prominent role. Water conducts heat 25 times faster than air!

Clothing is crucial to preventing hypothermia. Most of the insulating effect of clothing is due to the layers of air trapped in and around the clothing rather than to the insulating property of the clothing itself. Once water permeates the clothing, much of the insulation is lost. Nevertheless, even wet clothing has a surprisingly large effect on the overall rate of heat loss. It can reduce the rate of fall in core temperature by 50 to 75 percent. Water trapped beneath and in the interstices of the clothing conducts heat from the body. As its temperature rises, the trapped water acts as a buffer between the body and the cooler water in circulation. Water immediately surrounding the sailor is also warmed and acts as a weak heat buffer.

It should be obvious why swimming is so detrimental to cold water survival. First, it defeats the body's attempt to increase the size of the shell by pumping warm blood into the muscles. Second, swimming pumps out the already warmed layer of water within and beneath the clothing. Third, the water in the immediate proximity, which has been heated at the sailor's expense, is replaced with cold water. Unless the sailor is *absolutely certain* he can make it to a nearby object or to land, he is better off conserving his body heat. Remember the *Rule of 50s:*

50 yards in 50° F water = 50:50 chance

In fact, the sailor should avoid all exercise. It is now well established that the heat loss is invariably greater than the heat that can be generated by exercise in cold water. The first mate of the *Dancing Ledge* survived in spite of bicycling, not because of it!

If alone, the sailor should adopt the *heat escape lessening posture* (HELP) (Figure 2.5). This posture reduces heat loss from those areas that tend to lose heat the fastest: the head and neck, the sides of the chest, and the groin. The victim should lean back against the collar of the PFD,

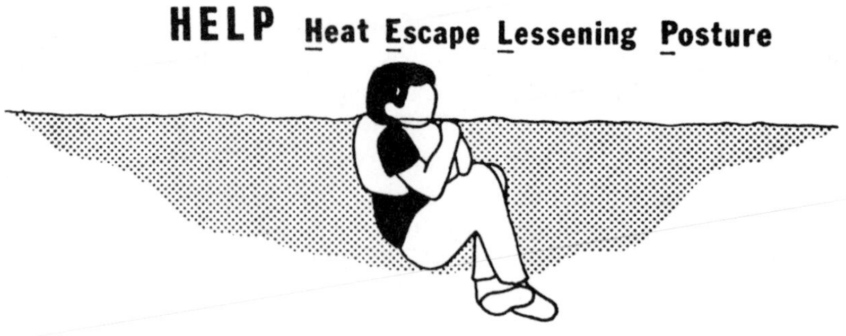

HELP   Heat Escape Lessening Posture

Figure 2.5. Heat escape lessening posture (HELP). Reprinted, by permission, from Robert S. Pratt, Hypothermia: The chill that need not kill, *American College of Surgeons,* Bulletin (*Chicago, October 1980*).

the arms drawing the PFD close to the body. The legs should be crossed below the knees. The older technique known as drownproofing, or the dead man's float, is no longer recommended. It consists of taking a deep breath and then allowing the head and arms to hang limply in the water, periodically raising the head above the water to take another breath. Although this maneuver conserves muscular energy, it allows a tremendous amount of heat to escape each time the head is submerged.

When two or more people are in the water, they should huddle together with their chests in contact and their arms and legs wrapped around each other (Figure 2.6). This position especially helps small children, who might perish quickly if left alone in the HELP position. Children already have a higher risk of developing hypothermia than adults since they have a greater surface area relative to their body weight from which to lose heat.

If the sailor is unsuccessful in his struggle to preserve body heat, he becomes hypothermic. Figure 2.7 illustrates the signs of progressive hypothermia. Notice how the use of a PFD prolongs survival time. In addition to providing some insulation, the PFD keeps the head out of the water. Otherwise, once confusion, disorientation, and semiconsciousness are present, the sailor drowns.

Initially, the victim of hypothermia is often quiet and reluctant to communicate. Judgment may be impaired, an important fact since it potentially imperils the safety of others. The victim may become confused, resistant to aid, and even combative. Movement is slow and uncoordinated. The combination of clumsiness and slurred speech make the victim appear drunk! Shivering is an important sign, but it cannot be relied upon. It may not be present if the individual must engage in demanding activity

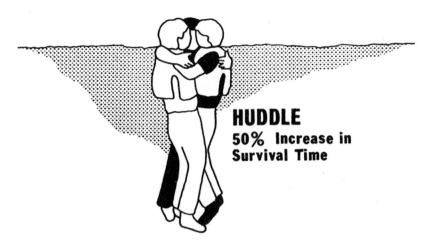

HUDDLE
50% Increase in
Survival Time

Figure 2.6. Huddle position for small groups. Reprinted, by permission, from Robert S. Pratt, Hypothermia: The chill that need not kill, *American College of Surgeons, Bulletin (Chicago, October 1980).*

(since exercise abolishes shivering), and as the core temperature declines, it is inevitably replaced by muscular rigidity.

When the core temperature drops to about 86° F (30° C), the sailor appears to be dead. There may be no sign of a pulse or of breathing. However, as the figure illustrates, appearances can be deceiving. Often a long period of time elapses during which the person seems to be dead but can still be revived. A medical rule for this particular situation states, "No one is dead unless they are warm and dead." Until the victim is warmed and still has no pulse or breathing, the rescuer should not forgo treatment. Once the core temperature has reached 77° F (25° C), the chances of successful revival become remote, although there are well-documented cases of people who have survived core temperatures below 68° F (20° C)!

If the victim is found with his head submerged in cold water, he may have activated the *mammalian diving reflex,* which will augment his chances for survival. This reflex occurs when the face (especially the area just above the bridge of the nose) is suddenly exposed to intense cold. The brain sets into motion a mechanism that rapidly reduces cardiac and respiratory activities to such a low level that they may not be discernible. This "instant hibernation," if you will, preserves the body for long periods of time and has been responsible for some of the dramatic recoveries reported from cold water drowning (so-called dry drownings). The mammalian diving reflex is independent of hypothermia, although they may coexist. The reflex is more likely to occur if the water is very cold and

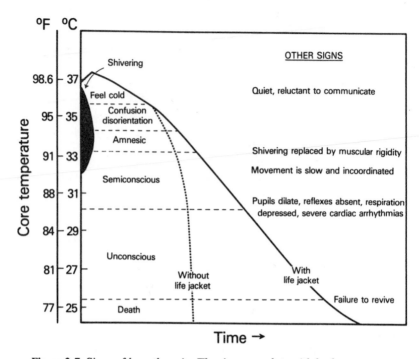

Figure 2.7. Signs of hypothermia. The signs correlate with body temperature, not with the time of immersion. The time at which these signs appear depends on many factors, such as the water temperature, duration of immersion, and the amount of clothing.

if the victim is young. Its incidence appears to decline as the age of the victim increases.

TREATMENT OF HYPOTHERMIA

If hypothermia is mild and the survivor is alert enough to recount his experiences (despite dramatic shivering), it is necessary only to remove his wet clothing and replace them with dry clothing or blankets. This treatment is known as *passive rewarming*. Sweetened, warm (but not hot) beverages such as cocoa should be given. Caffeine should be avoided initially and *in no case should the victim be given alcohol*. Alcohol has a number of deleterious effects: (1) it promotes heat loss, (2) it lowers blood sugar, and (3) it depresses the nervous system.

More severe cases require *active rewarming*. Hospital facilities have a number of means at their disposal for active rewarming, including those that selectively rewarm the core. Heat can be delivered by intravenous fluids, oxygen, dialysis, gastric lavage ("stomach pumping"), and even enemas; that is, *the victim can be warmed from the inside out.* If feasible, a victim who requires hospitalization should be prepared for evacuation at once. If the victim is semiconscious or unconscious, the first step is to transfer him *gently* to a warm environment. Unnecessary jostling must be avoided since it may precipitate fatal cardiac arrhythmias (irregularities) or cardiac arrest (cessation). His clothes should be removed with a minimum of movement—cut away if necessary—and his body should be covered to prevent further heat loss. The legs should be elevated to counteract the effects of shock, and the head should be kept slightly lower than the body to facilitate blood flow to the brain.

If there has been no pulse or breathing for 1 to 2 minutes (both of which, remember, may be slow and difficult to detect), a person who is properly trained should begin cardiopulmonary resuscitation (CPR). The reason to delay CPR with the hypothermic victim until there is definitely no pulse or breathing is that the procedure is a double-edged sword. Although it may be lifesaving, CPR may precipitate cardiac arrhythmia or arrest and so should be avoided unless absolutely necessary.

Active rewarming of the hypothermic victim *on the water* remains controversial. On the water, the only practical methods are immersion in a hot tub or shower, selective surface heating with hot packs or towels, and person-to-person contact (buddy warming). The drawback to each of these procedures is that *the victim is not warmed from the inside out but from the outside in.* As a result, the victim may experience a phenomenon known as afterdrop. In order to understand afterdrop, consider what would happen if we immersed the hypothermia victim in a tub of hot water. Since the arms and legs are part of the shell, they are maintained at a much lower temperature than the trunk by shunting blood away from them (see Figure 2.2). If the entire body is suddenly immersed in hot water, the blood vessels in the arms and legs will dilate and all of the "coldness" will flow back to the body core, cooling it further. This sudden return of cold blood may produce cardiac arrhythmias or arrest and is probably responsible for some of the fatalities that have occurred after initial recovery from hypothermia.

If tub immersion is attempted, the suggested temperature is 105° F to 110° F (40° C to 43° C), or slightly warmer if the victim is clothed. *It is imperative to keep the arms and legs out of the bath.* The temperature of the bath water will drop almost as soon as the victim is immersed so that hot water must be added frequently.

Probably the safest procedure for active rewarming on the water is to apply warm-to-hot wet towels or packs to the head, neck, chest, abdomen, and groin. Depending on their temperature, they will at least retard further heat loss and may provide some heat to the body. In conjunction, exhaling warm breath into the victim's face (in unison with his breathing) will supply some heat to the lungs, which are a part of the body core.

Person-to-person contact is readily accomplished. Both the victim and the volunteer must be naked, and contact should be restricted to the chest and back. A sleeping blanket is ideal for buddy warming.

Future research, it is hoped, will answer the question of whether or not active rewarming should be performed outside of the hospital. At present, all that can be said is that it is probably safe for young adults who have been hypothermic for brief periods of time. The alternative treatment, passive rewarming, is slow, laborious, and potentially ineffectual. The victim may not generate enough heat to rewarm himself, and the blankets may actually insulate him from the warmer environment.

KEEPING WARM ON THE WATER

In order to develop a sensible approach to keeping warm—instead of merely wearing whatever clothing is at hand—the sailor need only consider a few principles. The processes of heat exchange (radiation, conduction, evaporation, and convection) still operate with the addition of clothing, only now they are somewhat modified. Whereas clothing prevents radiation from the sun from reaching the body, it also intercepts radiation that the body is emitting into the environment. The net effect in a cold environment is to conserve body heat. Since clothing is in direct contact with the skin, some heat is lost via conduction. In practice, this loss is insignificant. Evaporation heat loss in the cold is the least-understood process. Although usually it too is negligible, in certain circumstances (discussed later in this chapter) a tremendous amount of heat may be lost via this route.

The most important avenue for heat loss is convection. Convection currents occur whenever there is a temperature gradient between the skin and the environment. Air that is heated through contact with the warmer skin rises to be replaced by cooler air (Figure 2.8). Thus, the body is constantly producing its own personal environment, or *microclimate,* of warm air. *The objective of all cold weather clothing is to preserve and augment this layer of warm air.*

Without clothing, convection currents inexorably play upon the skin,

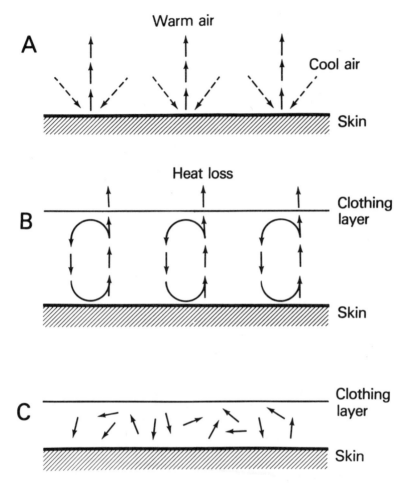

Figure 2.8. The influence of clothing on convection currents: (A) without clothing there is continual heat loss; (B) very loosely worn clothing allows circular convection currents to form; (C) optimal-layered clothing at approximately ¼-inch (6-millimeter) thickness prevents convection currents from forming.

draining heat from the body (Figure 2.8*A*). If the clothing is to be effective, it must control these currents. It may surprise you to learn that only a small percentage of the insulation clothing provides is due to the material itself. Most of the insulation is air trapped beneath and in the interstices of the garment and clinging in a layer to the garment's outer surface. Since air conducts heat very poorly, it is an exceptionally good insulating material. Keeping warm consists of utilizing the inherent insulating property of air!

Laboratory studies have shown that small laminations of "dead" air provide the best insulation for weight and flexibility (obviously important considerations to the sailor). This finding forms the basis of the "layer principle" that the armed forces have publicized so widely. The small laminations are most efficient at a thickness of approximately ¼ inch (6 millimeters). If the thickness of the dead air space is larger, the air rising on the warm side of the space (near the body) and settling along the cold side forms convection currents (Figure 2.8*B*). This circular motion rapidly increases heat loss. At ¼-inch thickness, there is enough air to provide insulation but not enough to create convection currents (Figure 2.8*C*). If the laminations of air become any smaller, the insulation is insufficient.

The crucial concept, of which many sailors are not cognizant, is that for the layer principle to be effective, the layers of clothing must be worn *loosely.* Otherwise the air is squeezed out from between the layers, and much of the insulation is lost. Thus, each additional layer should be sufficiently larger than the one before to allow for the thickness of the garment as well as for the thickness of the dead air space.[7] Unfortunately, as layers are built up on the body, a point of diminishing returns is reached. We can think of the body as being composed of variously shaped cylinders. As clothing is added, the surface area (from which heat is lost) of each of the cylinders increases. Eventually the increased surface area promotes more heat loss than the increased thickness can insulate. The fingers, as small cylinders, reach optimal insulation at about ¼ inch, whereas the trunk, a much larger cylinder, is still deriving insulation up to 5 or 6 inches. The arms and legs, moderate-size cylinders, benefit up to about 2 inches. The feet, each in reality a single cylinder of unusual shape since the toes tend to be cramped together, may be insulated to a thickness of ½ inch.

Sailors—and other outdoorsmen—tend to make the following mistakes:

1. The legs tend to be neglected. In fact they are larger cylinders than the arms and should have *more* insulation and not less, as is usually the case.

2. The arms tend to be overinsulated in comparison with the trunk. Since the trunk can profitably accommodate much thicker insulation than the arms, vests should be exploited to provide the additional trunk insulation.

3. The sailor whose feet are cold often incorrectly assumes that warmer footgear is the answer. Thicker footgear above the optimum will not improve matters. Rather, added insulation of the trunk may warm the feet. As the trunk is "overwarmed," some of this blood is shunted to the feet,

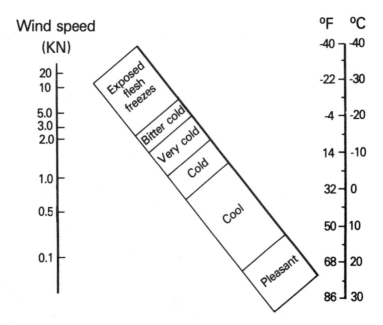

Figure 2.9. *Windchill factor. The subjective feeling of exposed flesh (such as face or hand) can be estimated with a straightedge. Line up the wind speed and the temperature. The intersection with the solid line in the center indicates the subjective feeling. For example, a temperature of 32° F (0° C) with a wind speed of 20 knots will be experienced as "very cold."*

from which heat escapes from the body. The feet act as heat radiators and keep themselves warm in the process.

To preserve the laminations of dead air, they must be protected from the wind. Thus a windbreaker is essential. By itself it provides an insignificant amount of insulation. However, by preserving the layers of dead air from the ravages of the wind, the windbreaker contributes enormously to the insulation process. It is foolish to go to the trouble of putting on layer upon layer of clothing to produce an "insulative edifice" without filling up the "chinks" to protect the layers from the wind. A windbreaker will also diminish the effect of the windchill factor, another misunderstood concept. Windchill is actually an estimate of the expected additional convection heat loss due to the wind. Since convection occurs most rapidly on exposed skin, the windchill factor (when stated in degrees of temperature) is strictly applicable to someone who is naked and exposed to the elements. It can accurately indicate, however, the subjective feeling of coldness over the exposed portions of the body such as the hands or face. Figure 2.9 is a simplified nomogram for calculating this subjective feeling. Notice that the left-hand scale for wind speed is "irregular"; that is, the rate of cooling is marked for the first few knots of wind, whereas the additional cooling produced by an increase from, say, 10 to 20 knots is rather modest. This makes sense if we recall that in the absence of any wind, convection currents produce a layer of warm air that surrounds the body. Although most of this warm air is beneath clothing when worn, the still air on the exterior is also warmed. As soon as the wind begins to blow (from 0.1 to 1 knot), this layer instantly vanishes. As the wind speed picks up, additional heat is lost, but at lesser increments.

The face and head have yet to be considered. These areas can be a significant source of heat loss—to such a degree that they have been likened to "a hole in a bucket." The face and head, unlike the rest of the body, do not undergo blood vessel constriction (vasoconstriction). On the contrary, the skin vasodilates, producing the familiar rosy red color so typical of cold weather.Thus a person usually suffers relatively little discomfort when exposing his face or entire head to very low temperatures. Unbeknown to him, heat from the rest of his body is rapidly flowing out from these areas. If at the same time he complains that his feet are cold, it may be more truth than jest that if he put on a hat, he would keep his feet warm! In other words, when the face and head are provided with protection—*even though they might not seem to need it*—more heat is retained in the body and warm blood is diverted to the feet, keeping them warm. A woolen cap can readily cover almost two-thirds of the head, and a thick "woolly" beard appreciably diminishes heat loss from the face.

Keeping warm also depends on choosing the right clothing materials. Many different measurements can be made to compare various materials. It turns out that *in still air* all fabrics provide about the same degree of insulation per inch of thickness. Is there any reason then for the universal preference for wool over other materials? The answer is yes, and the explanation lies in the structure of the wool. Wool is distinctive because of its natural crimp. There are 10 or more crimps, or undulations, per inch that impart a loftiness to the material, and this loftiness traps more air within the fibers. Natural wool also has microscopic surface scales that promote "aerodynamic drag," keeping the air in contact with the wool. Additional reasons for the superiority of wool are its elasticity and compressional resiliency, especially when moist. Dry cotton, for example, provides almost as much warmth as wool. But when moist, cotton loses its strength, is compressed, and consequently loses much of its insulative value. Wool tends to resist this compression better than the other natural or synthetic materials. However, synthetics that are spun to simulate wool perform almost as well as wool when wet, and they may dry faster and last longer!

Finally, in the effort to stay warm, there is one last requirement: clothing must have ventilation. The following case highlights this fact.

A soldier (a newcomer) was brought to the Fort Wainwright Hospital in a state of collapse during the 1965 Operation Polar Siege; he had been pulling sleds and chopping timber under conditions where the temperature was -40°. The diagnosis at the hospital was heat stroke. He had been so alarmed at the thought of working in the cold that he had piled on every item of insulation he could borrow.[8]

Thus, it is necessary to provide not only warmth but also flexibility for a wide range of conditions. This is particularly true for sailors since periods of intense (sometimes frantic) activity alternate with periods of relative inactivity. For example, by increasing exertion from that expended sitting on deck to that expended in light duty, the sailor approximately doubles his heat output and halves his insulation requirement. (This is not precisely correct, since some of the heat that exercise generates is lost.) Unless about half of the insulation is eliminated, sweating begins and *sweating must be avoided at all costs*. There are two alternatives: either some of the layers can be removed, or the whole "system" can be ventilated. The novice is generally reluctant to remove anything, whereas the old salt by habit avoids the danger of allowing sweat to accumulate in his clothing.

As soon as the sailor begins to feel hot, he should first remove his gloves and, if this is insufficient, his cap. Then, prior to removing layers, he should attempt to ventilate the system. The Eskimo, who are constantly confronted with an identical problem, have arrived at this very solution by designing fur clothing with vents that can be opened to permit controlled ventilation. When an Eskimo is stationary, he closes the apertures at the ankles, wrists, waist, and neck. As his level of activity increases, he opens these apertures, allowing upward ventilation through the neck region, so-called chimney ventilation. Most likely this was the original purpose of the necktie, with a knot that can be loosened without untying.

The reason that sweating must be avoided is that it is capable of promoting tremendous heat loss. It does this in two ways. First, there is a reduction in the amount of insulation. As the inner layers become wet, air is displaced from the fabric. Second, and even more important, the process of evaporation takes place. When the sailor begins to sweat, water vapor is produced at the skin surface. Body heat is required to produce the water vapor, and this heat is lost. But the process does not stop there. If the sailor is wearing waterproof foul-weather gear, the water vapor does not have ready access to the atmosphere. Despite manufacturers' claims that their newer waterproof fabrics can "breathe," these fabrics are still *relatively* impermeable to water vapor. In a short period of time, the inner layers become soggy. When the water vapor reaches the cooler, semi-impermeable wall of the foul-weather gear, it reaches dew point, and condensation takes place. Condensation liberates heat to the inner surface of the rain gear, and much of this heat is eventually lost. Gradually the entire space within the clothing layers reaches 100 percent humidity, and the liquid begins to soak backward. As it approaches the body surface, it is warmed and evaporates a second time, robbing the body of heat further. Once again it condenses on the inner surface of the rain gear. This cyclic process of evaporation and condensation accounts for the extreme cooling that occurs when damp clothes are worn under foul-weather gear.

The army has developed a mnemonic to assist their men in the proper use of clothing—COLD. The *C* is to remind the men to keep their clothing *clean* in order that it does not cling, become matted or greasy, and impair insulation; *O* suggests that the clothing be *opened* to avoid *overheating*; *L* recalls that clothing should be worn *loosely* and in *layers;* whereas *D* reminds them to keep the clothing *dry*.

Another piece of army advice that is applicable to the sailor is the use of "foxhole exercises." On a vessel, as in a foxhole, there is a limit to the amount and kind of exercise that can be performed to keep warm. The foxhole exercises consist of isometrically tensing successive groups of muscles. A person simply tenses the muscles of the neck, shoulders, arms, and hands sequentially until he has made a complete circuit of the body's muscles. It is not necessary to move visibly any portion of the body. The entire procedure can then be repeated several times. Previously cold hands and feet usually warm up in a few minutes, and the entire precedure may not be needed again for another half hour or hour.

PERFORMANCE IN THE COLD

There is one final caveat for the sailor who must function in a cold environment: he must anticipate that his efficiency will suffer. This results from the effect of cold on the muscles, nerves, and even the central nervous system if hypothermia is present.

Experiments conducted aboard ship reveal a deterioration in the ability to perform various tasks simultaneous with a fall in the skin temperature of the hand. The experiments tested handgrip strength and the ability to thread nuts onto screws and fasten screws into a metal plate—fairly representative of the kinds of tasks that a sailor might be called upon to perform. When the temperature of the skin fell below 60° F (15° C), there was a correspondent decline in both handgrip strength and manual dexterity. This decline cannot be attributed totally to the muscles. Many of the subjects also described difficulty in knowing what their fingers were doing! Subsequent experiments have confirmed that there is also a decrease in the sensation of the fingers at about 60° F (15° C). These effects are clearly the result of local cooling of the muscles and nerves. But what about the effects of cooling of the central nervous system (which is, after all, a part of the core)? Marked cooling produces the signs of hypothermia discussed earlier in this chapter (see Figure 2.5). Subtle cooling was evaluated in one experiment on watchkeeping proficiency in the wintertime. The test consisted of monitoring from the open bridge of a ship two lights separated by 75 degrees and signaling when a third, dimmer light appeared between the two. As a control, the test was repeated in a more temperate climate. In the cold, when the oral temperature (an approximation of the central core) fell as little as 1.2° F (0.7° C), there was a reliable increase in the number of delays in reporting the third light. Brain wave (electroencephalograph, or EEG) studies have also shown changes as soon as the core temperature cools as little as 2° F (1° C).

These findings have a number of implications for the sailor. When working in the cold, he should make allowance for diminished efficiency. He will require more time than previously for any given task, and, even if he has performed the task countless times before, he may need visual cues to compensate for the diminished finger dexterity and sensitivity. Finally, if exposure to the cold can be anticipated, it is advisable to dispense with the most complex tasks first before the inevitable decline occurs.

NOTES

1. There is no single "normal" temperature. Body temperature varies from one individual to another, as well as from one time of day to another for any given individual. It is usually highest at about 8 p.m. and lowest at about 5 a.m. The normal range for young healthy adults is 98° F to 100° F (36.7° C to 37.8° C) rectal or 97° F to 99° F (36.1° C to 37.2° C) oral.
2. D. Maclean and D. Emslie-Smith, *Accidental Hypothermia* (Oxford: Blackwell, 1977), p. 54.
3. R. H. Dana, *Two Years Before the Mast* (New York: Penguin, 1981), p. 393.
4. E. C. B. Lee and K. Lee, *Safety and Survival at Sea* (New York: Norton, 1980), p. 55.
5. K. A. Coles, *Heavy Weather Sailing,* Third revised edition, 1981 (Clinton Corners, N.Y.: De Graff, and London: Adlard Coles Ltd.), pp. 133-134.

6. The head is responsible for one-third of the body's heat loss. Putting on a cap, even if the foul-weather gear includes a hood, helps prolong survival time considerably.

Anyone who cruises extensively should consider one of the many survival suits. They increase survival time five- to tenfold. Although they are somewhat expensive, a case could be made that *not* having them is an example of false economy.

7. Norwegian fishnet underwear is worth considering as the initial layer. It serves two functions: maintaining a layer of dead air adjacent to the skin and keeping the subsequent layer off of the skin. By preventing the clothing from coming into contact with the skin, the fishnet diminishes the amount of moisture that is absorbed into the clothing, allowing more of the body moisture to pass through the clothing without wetting it.

8. G. E. Folk, *Introduction to Environmental Physiology* (Philadelphia: Lea & Febiger, 1966), p. 103.

3

Heat and Dehydration

Water, water every where,
And all the boards did shrink;
Water, water every where,
Nor any drop to drink.

S. T. Coleridge, *The Rime of the Ancient Mariner,* 1798

HEAT EXPOSURE PRESENTS THE sailor with just as severe a challenge as does exposure to the cold. The following account clearly demonstrates one of the most feared dangers—heatstroke:

> All the men lay spread on the uneven bundles of firewood blistering horribly in the tropical sun. Tongues began to blacken...and all vestiges of sanity deserted many.... One youngster, delirious with sunstroke, shouted the thoughts of his disordered mind for thirty hours before he became too weak to utter another word. Just before he died he grabbed a full tin, that was being used as a bed pan, and drank the contents greedily, before he could be prevented.[1]

In one respect, the challenge of heat exposure is even greater than that of the cold because there is less margin for error. As we saw in Chapter

TABLE 3.1
Normal Water Intake and Output for Adults

Intake (liters)		Output (liters)	
Water and beverages	1.2	Urine	1.3
Food water	0.9	Evaporation	1.0
Water of metabolism	0.4	Feces	0.2
	2.5		2.5

2, the normal core temperature is approximately 98.6° F (37° C). An average healthy adult may survive even when the core drops to 77° F (25° C), a decline of 21.6° F (12° C). Survival is rarely possible, however, if the core rises above 108° F (42° C), an elevation of only 9.4° F (5° C). Thus, over the range of core temperatures compatible with survival, the human "thermostat" is set high. The reason why this feature originally evolved will soon be evident.

Another crucial difference between heat and cold exposure is the body's requirement for water. The normal water intake and output for adults are shown in Table 3.1.

Food water refers to the water content of food. The water content of solid food is seldom less than 50 percent, and that of some fruits and vegetables may be as high as 90 percent. The amount of water produced during the metabolism of food (water of metabolism) depends on the type of food that is eaten. Fat yields the most water, carbohydrate somewhat less, and protein the least. This is one reason why the dehydrated sailor should avoid protein when water is scarce. There is another more important reason however. Fat and carbohydrate are metabolized into water and carbon dioxide (which the lungs excrete). The products of protein metabolism, primarily *urea*, the kidneys must excrete—and this process requires water. Thus fats and carbohydrates are preferred when water intake is low. The evaporation listed in the table refers to insensible water loss through the skin and from the lungs and *not* to the evaporation heat stress produces, which is frequently much larger. The water loss from feces, although of small magnitude, is important for normal evacuation. Its reduction during periods of dehydration is partially responsible for the common sailing malady of constipation.

In the cold, requirements for water are minimal. In a hot environment, the only means of eliminating heat—evaporation—is entirely dependent on water. Without water, evaporation fails, and without evaporation the sailor rapidly perishes.

EVAPORATION

Humans are most comfortable when they neither shiver nor sweat. The range between the two extremes is known as the thermoneutral zone and is roughly from 77° F (25° C) to 86° F (30° C). Below 77° F (25° C), either clothing or exercise is required to maintain body temperature. Without either, shivering will occur. Above 86° F (30° C) sweating begins. Within the thermoneutral zone, temperature regulation is most efficient. This process is carried out exclusively by the varying amount of blood flow to the skin, which determines the skin's thermal conductivity (see Figure 2.2). At the cool end of the thermoneutral zone, the superficial blood vessels are constricted, increasing the natural insulation of the skin and subcutaneous tissues. When the air temperature reaches 86° F (30° C), these vessels are fully dilated, promoting the transfer of heat from the core to the skin surface, where it can be eliminated.

When the blood vessels are fully dilated, heat dissipation by radiation and convection is at a maximal level, and evaporation must make up the difference. Once the air temperature rises above 95° F (35° C), the heat gradient reverses, and the body begins to *gain* heat by radiation and convection. *Evaporation is now the only means of eliminating heat from the body.* If any activity must be performed, evaporation must dispose of the heat generated from that as well. Fortunately, evaporation is capable of eliminating tremendous amounts of heat.

Dr. Charles Blagden first demonstrated the remarkable capacity of evaporation 200 years ago.[2] He, along with a few friends and a dog, entered a room heated to 260° F (120° C). They remained in the room for 45 minutes without ill effects, while the beefsteak they brought in with them was thoroughly cooked in 15 minutes. More recent experiments have confirmed his observations. For short periods of time, man can produce sweat at a rate of 4 quarts (about 4 liters) per hour! The magnitude of this accomplishment can be appreciated when we recall that an adult has only 5 quarts (about 5 liters) of circulating blood at any one time. Obviously there is a price to pay for this kind of energy efficiency, and it is paid in salt and water—especially water.

SWEAT

The human body is endowed with two different kinds of sweat glands. The *apocrine* glands are located in the axillary, mammary, and pubic

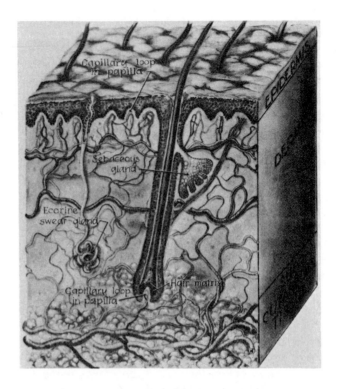

Figure 3.1. Cross section of the skin. Reproduced, by permission, from D. M. Pillsbury and C. L. Heaton, A Manual of Dermatology, *2d ed. (Philadelphia: W. B. Saunders, 1980).*

regions. They function primarily in sex and reproduction, not in temperature regulation. In the average adult there are 2 million to 4 million *eccrine* glands concentrated in certain regions of the body. Sweat is most copious from these regions. The highest concentration (and hence the greatest sweating) occurs on the forehead, neck, trunk, and back of the hand. Lesser degrees of sweating occur on the cheeks and the remainder on the arms and legs. The underarms, palms, and soles sweat the least in the heat, in contrast to their production under psychological stress. The eccrine glands lie deep in the skin and are connected to the surface by twisted coils (Figure 3.1). When blood passes through the glands, water and salt are extracted and secreted. At the skin surface the sweat evaporates, liberating heat from the body. *Sweating per se does nothing to cool the body. For heat to be liberated, the sweat must undergo evaporation at the skin surface. Sweat that drips from the skin without evaporating is entirely wasted.* The efficiency of evaporation is ultimately determined by the degree of atmospheric humidity. During periods of high humidity, the air is already holding a great deal of water, limiting evaporation from the skin.

Although the ability to sweat is taken for granted, there is a marked variation from one individual to another. Some people are able to produce sweat at a rate of 4 quarts (4 liters) per hour for brief periods of time, whereas others are capable of only a meager pint (0.5 liter) under the same conditions. Rare individuals are unable to sweat at all. This variation in sweating ability explains in part why certain individuals are more susceptible than others to some of the heat-induced disorders, such as heatstroke. Skin disorders such as prickly heat or rash interfere with sweating, as do a number of widely prescribed drugs, including many of those used to treat nervous and mental conditions (Table 3.2).

If there is a plentiful supply of water (and salt), a person can survive long periods of intense heat. In fact, with daily exposure he begins to acclimatize in 4 days and is fully adapted to the heat in about a week. Acclimatization improves the overall efficiency of the system. The threshold for sweating is lower, and the sweat is distributed more uniformly over the body, which promotes evaporation. In addition, body temperature and heart rate, which were initially elevated, return to normal.

It is worth noting that during an initial exposure to a hot environment, the body has a tendency to become dehydrated even when salt and water are freely available. This common phenomenon is known as voluntary dehydration. For some reason, thirst is often satisfied before all of the salt and water have been replaced. Therefore, if supplies are plentiful, the sailor should be encouraged to drink and replace his salt liberally.

When water is scarce, a problem most shipwreck survivors face, the sailor is in danger of becoming progressively dehydrated. It is logical to assume that the rate of sweating would decline with progressive dehydration, but in fact the decrease is slight. By and large, sweating continues at a rate determined by the temperature, rather than the degree of dehydration. The sailor is clearly "between a rock and a hard place." If, on the one hand, sweating is reduced to preserve body water, body heat rises to unacceptable levels. If, on the other hand, sweating continues, the sailor becomes increasingly dehydrated. Since the effect of uncontrolled heat gain has a fatal effect more rapidly than dehydration, there is little choice but to accept a substantial amount of dehydration.

The sailor tolerates well a certain amount of dehydration, giving him time to search for sources of water. However, once the water deficit approaches 10 percent of body weight, the system begins to falter. Core

TABLE 3.2
Drugs That Can Interfere with Sweating*

Major Tranquilizers

chlorpromazine *(Thorazine)*   trifluoperazine *(Stelazine)*
thioridazine *(Mellaril)*   haloperidol *(Haldol)*
perphenazine *(Trilafon)*   thiothixene *(Navane)*
promazine *(Sparine)*   loxapine *(Loxitane)*
triflupromazine *(Vesprin)*   molindone *(Moban)*
fluphenazine *(Prolixin)*

Antidepressants

amitriptyline *(Elavil)*   maprotiline *(Ludiomil)*
doxepin *(Sinequan)*   amoxapine *(Asendin)*
nortriptyline *(Aventyl)*   tranylcypromine *(Parnate)*
imipramine *(Tofranil)*   isocarboxazid *(Marplan)*
protriptyline *(Vivactil)*   pargyline *(Eutonyl)*
desipramine *(Norpramin)*   phenelzine *(Nardil)*
lithium *(Eskalith)*

Drugs Used to Treat Parkinson's Disease

trihexyphenidyl *(Artane)*
benztropine *(Cogentin)*
biperiden *(Akineton)*

Drugs Used to Treat Abdominal Upset

prochlorperazine *(Compazine)*
belladonna alkaloids *(Donnatal) (Bellergal)*

Some Antihistamines

diphenhydramine *(Benadryl)*
hydroxyzine *(Vistaril) (Atarax)*

*Note: This list is only representative of the kinds of drugs that can interfere
with sweating. Most of the severe reactions have been attributed to the major
tranquilizers. If you are not certain about a particular drug, check with your
physician or pharmacist. See Appendix for common drug equivalents.*

temperature is now about 102° F (39° C). The reduction in the blood
volume due to the water loss compromises the heart and circulatory system.
In addition, the viscosity of the blood increases, further taxing the system.
If water is not available soon, the sailor will die of dehydration.

The degree of dehydration can be estimated as follows: at 2 percent weight loss, there is appreciable thirst; at 4 percent, the mouth and throat are exceedingly dry; at 8 percent, salivation stops and speech becomes difficult; at 10 percent, the sailor is unable to care for himself; at 12 percent, he is unable to swallow and will recover only if water is given by stomach tube, rectal enema, or intravenously. It is unknown at what point sweating fails, but in humans it is probably at about 18 to 20 percent.

We can now make a guess at why our thermostat is set on the high side. If our body temperature were set at, say, 86° F (30° C), it would not be physically possible to produce enough sweat fast enough to cool ourselves at an air temperature of only 100° F (38° C)! With the thermostat set high, the onset of our efficient but costly evaporative cooling system is delayed as long as possible.

Not only is there a substantial loss of water in dehydration, but a significant amount of salt loss as well. The body normally contains an estimated 160 grams of salt, the most important of which is sodium chloride, or table salt. The body is also rich in other salts such as potassium and magnesium, but since only sodium chloride is lost in large quantities in sweat, the others can be temporarily neglected. The *concentration* of salts in the body is just as important as—and sometimes more important than—the total quantity. The kidneys, the major arbiter of our internal environment, maintain this concentration within narrow limits at approximately a 0.9 percent solution.

Under normal circumstances if we ingest an excess amount of salt, three things usually occur. The increased salt concentration stimulates the thirst mechanism, we increase water intake, and with this water the kidneys excrete the excess salt in the urine, reestablishing a 0.9 percent solution. If there is a deficiency of salt, however, the kidneys jealously conserve what is left by decreasing the amount of salt in the urine.

Not only is the rate of sweating variable, but so is the concentration of salt in sweat. The average concentration is 0.2 to 0.3 percent, with a range of 0.1 to 0.6 percent. In a very hot environment, the body, especially if under physical stress, usually begins to excrete sweat with a salt concentration of about 0.45 percent—about half the concentration in blood. Sweating rates of 5 to 7 quarts (5 to 7 liters) per day—and 8 to 12 quarts (8 to 12 liters) per day are possible—produce a salt deficit of about 20 to 25 grams, a loss of over 15 percent! Clearly something must be done to reduce the amount of salt loss. The kidneys respond immediately by curtailing urinary salt altogether. In addition, over the next few days the concentration of salt in the sweat is reduced. By this time, however, the sailor already has a significant deficit in salt and water.

Ideally, salt and water should be replaced at the same rate and concentration at which they were lost in the sweat. Unfortunately, there is no easy way to determine such losses at sea. A practical approach to take is as follows: *If water is readily available,* the amount of salt in the diet should be increased from 10 grams to 20 to 25 grams per day. Slightly less is necessary if sweating is not profuse. This measure will satisfy the needs of all but the rare few who secrete a very concentrated sweat. Some of the salt can be replaced in the food (cooking and table salt), whereas the rest can be replenished with salt tablets, which are often 1 gram each.[3] Potassium supplements are usually not needed because the potassium loss in sweat is small. Anyway, a glass of orange or tomato juice replaces nearly all of the potassium, calcium, and magnesium excreted in about 3 quarts (3 liters) of sweat. There is no need to worry about overdose. In healthy adults the kidneys easily excrete any excess salt. *If water is not readily available,* as in shipwreck situations, salt should be avoided. The reason is that even the most concentrated sweat is less concentrated than normal body tissues (0.9 percent), so the shipwrecked sailor with a limited water supply will always be more deficient in water than salt. Only when he has replaced the water should he take salt.

HEAT-INDUCED DISORDERS

A common heat-induced disorder is *heat cramps.* Although quite painful, the condition is fortunately nearly always benign. Sir Francis Chichester describes it in *Gipsy Moth Circles the World:*

> I don't get hungry in these 85° F heats until the middle of the night, or early morning.... At night I was troubled by cramp in my legs which would hit me after I had been asleep about two hours, and would let go only if I stood up. This meant that I never got more than about two hours sleep at a time. It was hot and I sweated profusely; I wondered whether my body might be losing too much salt. I decided to drink half a glassful of sea-water a day to put back salt.[4]

The cramps begin suddenly and most frequently attack the legs and thighs, although they may also affect the abdomen, arms, hands, feet, or even the jaw. They last for hours at a time and continue until the salt deficiency is corrected. The cramps usually afflict the sailor who has been drinking large amounts of fluids without replenishing the salt.

Heat cramps may occur alone or as part of the disorder known as *heat exhaustion.* Heat exhaustion can be mild or severe. Mild heat exhaustion (also known as heat collapse, or heat syncope) occurs in the unacclimatized sailor. He experiences progressive lassitude and is unable to work. Par-

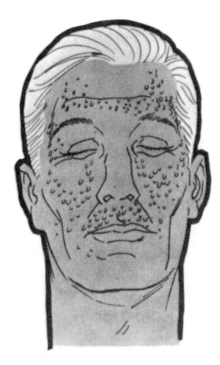

Figure 3.2. Heat exhaustion.

tially responsible is a salt *and* water deficiency, which temporarily diminishes the amount of blood circulating in the body. In addition, heat dilates the capillaries of the skin, allowing blood to pool there, further diminishing the amount of blood that the heart can pump to the rest of the body. Sudden changes in posture, such as rising quickly, result in dizziness and passing out.

The severe form occurs with more extreme degrees of salt deficiency. In the absence of salt, water that is ingested does not replenish the blood supply but is excreted in the urine to maintain the proper salt concentration (0.9 percent). In other words, *the blood volume can never be fully replenished until the salt is replaced.* The symptoms of severe heat exhaustion resemble those of shock and in rare cases may be lethal. The pulse is rapid and weak, blood pressure is low, and there is weakness, dizziness, headache, nausea, and blurred vision. In both forms of heat exhaustion, body temperature may be normal, subnormal, or slightly elevated. Sweating is profuse (Figure 3.2). The treatment requires an increase in dietary salt and water.

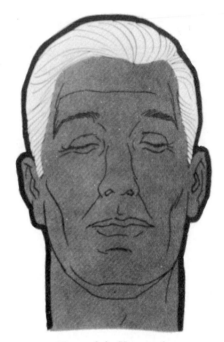

Figure 3.3. Heatstroke.

Whereas heat exhaustion is the end result of a normal, functioning temperature-regulating system, *heatstroke* occurs when this system fails. Heatstroke is easily distinguished from heat exhaustion by the total absence of sweating. The sailor's skin is red, hot, and bone dry (Figure 3.3). Usually sweating ceases completely, and the temperature rises to 104° F (40° C) or higher. Periods of delirium (as described in the excerpt at the beginning of the chapter) are quite common, as are convulsive seizures and eventually coma.

Although heatstroke may occur with dramatic suddenness (hence the term *stroke*), it is often preceded by numerous warning symptoms, such as faintness, headache, staggering, and brief episodes of mental confusion. A few sailors have noticed that their sweating capacity has declined in the days prior to heatstroke. Unfortunately, this important warning is invariably neglected. *It is vital to recognize the early warning signs of heatstroke because the mortality rate is as high as 50 percent!* Even if the individual survives, he may sustain permanent damage to the brain, heart, kidneys, or liver.

The cause of heatstroke is still unknown. It has commonly been attributed to "sweat-gland fatigue," but since sweating fails all at once over the entire body, this seems unlikely. More likely the central temperature-regulating system, which is located in the hypothalamic region of the brain, is damaged, and sweating is inappropriately "turned off."[5]

Although the cause is unknown, some factors seem to predispose to its development, including poor overall health, increasing age, obesity, lack of acclimatization, extensive prickly heat or other skin diseases, alcohol, and drugs that inhibit sweating (Table 3.2). Previous, even mild, episodes of heatstroke are the most serious predisposing factor. They may disrupt the temperature-regulation system and inhibit sweating for months or years afterward. Occasionally the inability to sweat is permanent!

The treatment of heatstroke consists of reducing the body temperature as rapidly as possible. The sailor should be undressed and placed in a tub of ice water. If that is not feasible, he should be covered with ice packs or sponged with cold water until his temperature drops. The skin should be massaged vigorously at this time to prevent constriction of the blood vessels of the skin (due to the cold water) and to stimulate the return of cool blood to the body core. After the body temperature has dropped, the victim should be placed in a cold room or the coolest place on the boat. If the body temperature starts to rise again, it will be necessary to repeat the cooling procedure. The sailor should be kept in bed for several days after an episode of heatstroke and should avoid heat exposure for some time.

HEAT AND THE HYPERTENSIVE SAILOR

Any sailor who has a diagnosis of hypertension (high blood pressure) must exercise particular caution in the heat. Most hypertensive individuals are kept on a low-sodium diet, which, of course, restricts salt intake. This produces a dilemma. If the sailor reduces his salt intake, he will become more susceptible to the heat-induced disorders described above. Yet if he increases his salt intake to compensate for his losses, he may aggravate his hypertension. There is no simple solution. The sailor may circumvent the problem, however, if he pays special attention to his rate of sweating and attempts to replace only his losses. He cannot be quite as liberal in his salt replacement as can his nonhypertensive mate.

The hypertensive sailor may have to face an additional dilemma. If he is being treated with a diuretic, or "fluid pill" (the medication of choice for certain types of hypertension), his tolerance to heat is even less, since he is already slightly dehydrated before he even begins to sweat. Some physicians try to compensate by prescribing a slightly lower dose of diuretic for those patients who will be exposed to intense heat. However, this is hardly a satisfactory solution to the problem.

PERFORMANCE IN THE HEAT

Studies of human performance in the heat are not as clear-cut as those of performance in the cold. In fact, despite numerous experiments conducted over three decades, the results remain somewhat contradictory. Nevertheless, they have revealed one important distinction between performance in a hot environment and in a cold environment. Even in the absence of a lowered core temperature (i.e., hypothermia), a cold environment reduces the function of exposed arms and legs; that is, cold "slows down" the muscles and nerves (both sensory and motor). This does not occur in the heat. A hot environment has little direct effect on either muscles or nerves.

Impairment of human performance in the heat therefore occurs only with the rise of deep body temperature. No matter how great the heat load, the sailor is able to function at, or very nearly at, his usual level until his body temperature begins to rise. Once this occurs, his ability to perform the most complex tasks deteriorates. Simple tasks such as visual tracking suffer next. His performance of primarily mental tasks remains *relatively* unimpaired until close to the endurance level.

SURVIVAL

An altogether different problem confronts the sailor who is forced to abandon ship—a restricted supply of water. In one sense there is never a shortage of water in a marine environment—only a shortage of *potable* water. The high salt content, or salinity, of seawater generally prohibits its consumption.

The salinity of seawater varies little around the globe. It ranges from a 3.5 to a 3.7 percent solution, except in the Mediterranean and the Red Sea where it is slightly higher (3.7 to 4.1 percent). This 3.5 percent solution consists of primarily sodium chloride (2.8 to 3.0 percent), as well as smaller amounts of such salts as calcium chloride, magnesium chloride, magnesium sulfate, and potassium chloride.

Animals have established an accommodation with nature and are able to extract water from the "hostile" environment. Most species of saltwater fish simply excrete excess salt through their gills directly back into the ocean. Oceanic birds such as the cormorant, pelican, and albatross are able to tolerate drinking seawater by excreting most of the ingested salt through specially developed salt glands (nasal glands). Since this salt solution is more concentrated than seawater, the birds end up with a net gain in water. Whales, dolphins, and seals have adopted a different strategy altogether. These animals obtain virtually all of their water from the metabolism of food, particularly fat. There is no evidence that they can tolerate seawater any better than we can. Other animals, especially some desert-dwelling mammals that are in constant need of water, possess kidneys of great concentrating power. The kangaroo rat, for example, excretes a urine that is four times as concentrated as is man's. This animal can thrive on a diet of seawater.[6]

How much water is necessary for man to survive? Obviously, the requirements vary with the climatic conditions and the amount of work that must be done. With no water whatsoever, the following survival times may be expected. They are rough approximations based on *mean air temperature,* which takes into account the lower nighttime temperature at sea:

98.6° F (37° C)	—	2 days
89.6° F (32° C)	—	3 days
78.8° F (26° C)	—	4 days
69.8° F (21° C)	—	8 days
59.0° F (15° C)	—	10 days

These figures are applicable to a sailor who does not have to perform an appreciable amount of work. Hard work requires more water. According to previous dogma, 1 pint (0.5 liter) per day was required to sustain a man for longer periods of time. However, recent survival accounts indicate that this figure can probably be revised downward to about 0.33 pint (0.16 liter) per day (see the discussion on the Robertsons and the Baileys later in this chapter).

Many sources of water are available to the shipwreck survivor. These can be divided into *freshwater* sources (which are preferred) and *other* sources. There are only four sources of fresh water: (1) water rations stored in or brought aboard the survival craft, (2) rainwater, (3) water that has been chemically desalinated, and (4) water produced in a solar distillation unit, or "solar still."

It is ironic that solar stills have not played a greater role in recent survival stories since a method of distillation was used at sea in Elizabethan times. Sir Richard Hawkins in his *Observations on a Voyage to the South Seas* reported:

> Although our fresh water had fayled us many days before we saw the shore, by reason of our long navigation and the excessive drinking of the sicke and the diseased, yet with an invention I had in my shippe, I easily drew out of the water of the sea sufficient quantity of fresh water to sustain my people, with little expense of fewell [fuel]; for with foure billets [of wood] I stilled a hogshead [over 63 gallons] of water and therewith dressed the meat for the sicke and whole. The water so distilled we found wholesome and nourishing.[7]

Although solar stills are a bit tricky to use and are currently limited in output to about 1 quart (l liter) per day (depending on the latitude), one or more should be aboard *every* life raft.

Water can be coaxed from other sources in the environment, including the tissues of marine creatures such as fish, sea turtles, and marine birds. Two splendid discussions of these sources are *Survive the Savage Sea,* by Dougal Robertson, and *Staying Alive,* by Maurice and Maralyn Bailey.[8] Since the Robertsons were in worse shape in regard to water stores, let us examine their story.

Robertson, his wife (a nurse), and four children were shipwrecked when killer whales attacked their schooner west of the Galapagos Islands on June 15, 1972. The boat sank in 60 seconds, leaving little time for coordinated preparation. They survived and were subsequently rescued from their dinghy 38 days later, although it seems likely that they would soon have made a landing on the coast of Costa Rica. Their survival (and that of the Baileys, who survived 117 days in virtually the same region of the Pacific) is a testament to man's ability to wrest sustenance, especially water, from the sea. The Robertsons were equipped with emergency rations of food and water for only 3 days and lived almost entirely on rainwater and marine life.

Rainwater was their most highly prized commodity, and with Robertson's ingenuity they were able to use almost all of it. Because of the improvisational nature of their rain-catching system, the initial part of the collection, although technically *potable,* was not *palatable.* This portion was separated from the rest and given via a plastic tube as a water-retention enema. Up to 1 pint (0.5 liter) of water can be readily absorbed in this fashion. As his wife pointed out, this technique is only effective for unpalatable fresh water, not seawater. Seawater given via retention enema causes just as much havoc as it would if taken orally.[9]

Sea turtles and fish were the mainstays of their existence. Each 75-pound (34-kilogram) turtle yields 3 to 4 pints (1.5 to 2 liters) of blood. The blood coagulates in about a minute, so it must be drunk immediately. The cerebrospinal fluid from the spinal cavity and the eyeball fluid, although limited in quantity, are even purer sources of water (lower salinity). These fluids can be obtained from turtles, fish, and even marine birds! Both the Robertsons and the Baileys utilized them. Curiously, neither of these authors mentions extracting "fish juice" (see the discussion later in this chapter).

The metabolism of food also produces water. As discussed earlier in this chapter, either fat or carbohydrate is superior to protein. According to classical teaching, it is best to avoid protein when less than 2 pints (1 liter) of water is available, although Robertson suggests that small amounts of protein can be eaten with somewhat less water than this. Nevertheless, if there is a choice, fat or carbohydrate is preferable.

In maintaining fluid balance, it is equally important to reduce the losses. The output of urine is already reduced to a minimum, and nothing further can be done. Some water continues to be lost via evaporation from the lungs, but it is relatively insignificant. What is significant is sweating. The sailor should take every opportunity during the day to keep his body as cool as possible. Keeping out of the sun is most important. Robertson states, "The double canopy alone was worth a gallon [4 liters] of water a day to us in keeping out the heat of the sun."[10] Strenuous work should be done at night if possible. The Baileys, during the early days of their ordeal, decided to try to row to safety. They realized that this could only be done at night. Brief baths in the ocean are possible, but the sailor must be careful to avoid the twin dangers of sharks and separation from the craft. Cool-water compresses and wrapping portions of the body with cool, wet cloths can be tried. The sailor should avoid overdoing it, however, since constant contact of the skin with seawater has a tendency to produce boils, which are quite painful. Continuous immersion eventually causes the skin to break down. Once this happens, the sailor is in serious trouble, since water losses increase tremendously in the presence of denuded skin.

Finally, it should be noted that the Robertsons survived for 7 days on as little as 0.33 pint (0.16 liter) per day and, except for brief respites, the remainder of their ordeal with 1 pint (0.5 liter) or less per day! This experience, and others like it, should be kept in mind when considering the seawater controversy.[11]

THE SEAWATER CONTROVERSY

The controversy over whether or not the castaway should ever drink seawater seems destined to be with us for some time. What probably keeps it alive is the supreme irony of suffering and dying from thirst while surrounded by water. Actually, the controversy is a lopsided affair. On one side is the Goliath of international medical opinion. The British Department of Trade clearly summarizes this position:

> Seafarers are reminded that if cast away they should *never under any circumstances drink sea water* which has not been through a distillation plant, or de-salinated by chemical means. A belief has arisen that it is possible to replace or supplement fresh water rations by drinking sea water in small amounts. This belief is wrong and *dangerous.*
>
> Drinking untreated sea water does a thirsty man no good at all. It will lead to increased dehydration and thirst and may kill him.
>
> Even if there is no fresh water at all it should be remembered that men have lived for many days with nothing to drink, and therefore the temptation to drink untreated sea water must be strongly resisted.[12]

Dr. Alain Bombard, a feisty French physician, plays the role of David in this affair. In 1952 Bombard, recently out of medical school, decided to prove that man could live entirely on the sustenance the sea provided and so became a "voluntary castaway." He spent 65 days at sea in an inflatable life raft traveling from Las Palmas in the Canary Islands to Barbados without relying on supplies of food or water. Apparently, his only water for the first 24 days at sea consisted of seawater and fish juice. After this period, squalls were frequent enough to provide a reserve of fresh water.

His position about the use of seawater is still sometimes misunderstood. He does *not* advocate its use in the face of dehydration. Everyone is in agreement that once the survivor is seriously dehydrated, drinking seawater is extremely dangerous. What he does advocate is the *early* use of seawater to supplement or extend the freshwater supply. If absolutely no fresh water is available, he suggests small amounts of seawater as a stopgap measure until something better turns up. He argues that even though drinking seawater increases the rate of dehydration, it gives the castaway additional time to find other sources. If the supply of fresh water is limited—as is usually the case—he advocates mixing it with seawater in a ratio of two to one (two parts fresh water to one part seawater).

In order to appreciate both the risks and the potential benefits of drinking seawater, let us first examine a situation in which the use of seawater is indisputably contraindicated—the case of the severely dehydrated survivor.

The normal salinity of most human and animal body fluids is about 0.9 percent. Any fluid that has this concentration of dissolved salts is referred to as *isotonic*. Seawater (3.5 percent) has almost four times as much dissolved salt and so is *hypertonic.* A liquid that is less concentrated than 0.9 percent is *hypotonic.* Pure fresh water is as hypotonic as you can get.

In every instance, the dehydrated sailor, although deficient in both salt and water, will be much more deficient in water. This causes the concentration of salt in the body to be higher than normal—a condition known as hypernatremia. What if the sailor now drinks seawater? Under the best of circumstances, the kidneys are able to excrete a urine almost as concentrated as seawater. However, salt accounts for only a little more than half of the dissolved substances in the urine, approximately a 1.5 percent solution. The other half is practically all urea, the main end product of protein metabolism. Thus, if the sailor drinks a 3.5 percent solution and is able to excrete only a 1.5 percent solution, he will end up with a net loss of water. In addition, if the urine is to remain maximally concentrated, the kidneys can only deal with small amounts of dissolved substances. If the kidneys have to get rid of large amounts of dissolved substances—either salt after the drinking of seawater or urea after a large protein meal—they are no longer capable of producing a maximally concentrated urine. In other words, the more salt the kidneys have to excrete, the lower the concentration and the greater the net loss of water.

The increasing salt concentration in the body (hypernatremia) has drastic consequences including delirium, hallucinations, epileptic convulsions, coma, and death.

> Many of the crew drank sea water; although I threatened to stop their fresh water if they continued to do so, many of the men continued to drink it at night; I could always tell when a man had been drinking salt water because the guilty ones suffered from hallucinations. During the tenth day the second cook became insane probably through drinking of sea water.[13]

What about drinking straight seawater soon after shipwreck, perhaps two to three mouthfuls every 3 hours? This is also a bad idea. Since the sailor is not yet deficient in either salt or water, *all* of the salt will have to be excreted, thereby increasing again the rate of dehydration. He is better off having nothing than having straight seawater.

If the survivor has some fresh water, should he attempt to extend it by mixing it with seawater? Probably not, but this is where the waters become murky. We must keep in mind the distinction between what the body can tolerate and what is beneficial. There is no question that the body can tolerate dilute salt solutions—the more dilute or hypotonic the better. If we dilute in a ratio of 2 to 1, the concentration is reduced to about 1.2 percent, below the kidneys' maximum of about 1.5 percent. But we must remember the kidneys excrete 1.5 percent only if there is not too much salt to contend with. To be safe, it is best to dilute in a ratio of 3 to 1 or more. A 3-to-1 dilution produces an isotonic (0.9 percent) solution. However, since the average concentration of sweat is only 0.2 to 0.3 percent, the sailor, to replace his losses with seawater, ideally should dilute at about 10 to 1.

One problem is obvious. The more the sailor dilutes, the less he is going to extend his freshwater supplies. It's just not worth it. But there is another, more dangerous problem: establishing a precedent of drinking seawater in the first place. Robertson addresses just this point:

> Since the castaway has to adopt some personal attitude to this argument perhaps our experience can be of some assistance to him in arriving at a decision. All evidence, from both sides of the argument, points to the fact that if the body of the survivor is at all dehydrated, sea water can not only cause damage to internal organs and sickness, but it will intensify the dehydrated condition. Most advocates of the sea-water theory qualify their advocacy by stating that it can only be usefully assimilated by a body that doesn't really need it. During periods of severe thirst when we were on raft and dinghy, Lyn [his wife] and Douglas [a son] both admitted to an almost overwhelming desire to drink sea water, both by day and night. Only their own moral fiber prevented them from doing so, but how much would that moral fiber have been weakened if they had drunk some sea water in the initial stages after the disaster?[14]

Instead of posing the question, "Should I, or should I not, drink seawater?" it would probably be better to rank according to potability all of the possible sources of water available (Table 3.3). This approach avoids classifying seawater as a "poison," as well as discarding fresh water that has been adulterated with it. The Baileys apparently made this error when on their second day they discovered that 4 gallons (16 liters), or 40 percent, of their water supply had been contaminated with seawater. Since the water containers were presumably almost full at the time, it is likely that the adulterated water would still have been quite useful.

How can one estimate the salinity? The only rule of thumb is that if a fluid tastes salty, its concentration is probably 0.9 percent or greater. This is about the threshold for the appreciation of salt. But as the sailor becomes dehydrated and his salt concentration rises, his threshold also rises. This phenomenon explains why blood tastes a bit salty to people under normal conditions, but not at all to the dehydrated sailor!

Although there is some variation from species to species, the fluids and tissues of most marine animals are approximately isotonic. Fish juice (the fluid drained or squeezed from the body of a freshly caught fish) and sea turtle blood are good examples of isotonic marine fluids that can be util-

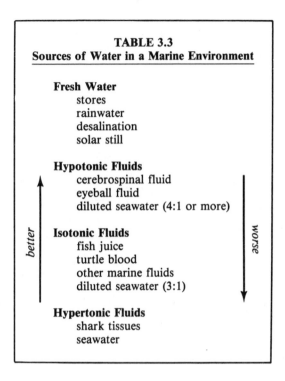

TABLE 3.3
Sources of Water in a Marine Environment

Fresh Water
stores
rainwater
desalination
solar still

Hypotonic Fluids
cerebrospinal fluid
eyeball fluid
diluted seawater (4:1 or more)

Isotonic Fluids
fish juice
turtle blood
other marine fluids
diluted seawater (3:1)

Hypertonic Fluids
shark tissues
seawater

better

worse

ized. Surgeon Captain J. D. Walters states that some species of turtles have hypotonic blood.[15] So much the better: hypotonic fluids are clearly superior. The cerebrospinal fluid of fish and turtles is hypotonic, as is man's. The same applies to eyeball fluid. Although both of these sources are small, in survival situations, all sources become important.

One animal should be avoided unless there is plenty of water available—the shark. Both the Robertsons and the Baileys caught small sharks. The sharks (and related species) are unique in that they have a tissue concentration that is the same as seawater! They achieve their 3.5 percent concentration not with salt but with urea, which is present in enormous quantities. Because the kidneys must excrete urea directly, it tends to produce dehydration just as much as seawater.

NOTES

1. E. C. B. Lee and K. Lee, *Safety and Survival at Sea* (New York: W.W. Norton, 1980), p. 90.

2. C. Blagden, "Further Experiments and Observations in a Heated Room," in *Phil. Trans. Roy. Soc. Lond.* 65 (1775): 484-494.

3. Some individuals find it difficult to tolerate salt tablets because of nausea and vomiting.

4. Sir Francis Chichester, *Gipsy Moth Circles the World* (London: Hodder & Stoughton, and New York: Coward-McCann, 1967), p. 46.

5. Contrary to the classical view that heatstroke is due to a breakdown of the heat-dissipation mechanism causing a cessation of sweating, some recent evidence suggests that the primary factor may be an excessively high core temperature. This would explain the uncommon occurrence of heatstroke in the presence of profuse sweating.

6. The different lifestyles that have evolved in response to the ever-present need to preserve salt and water are beyond the scope of this chapter. The reader is referred to the works of Homer W. Smith, in particular the classic *From Fish to Philosopher* (Garden City, N.Y.: Anchor, 1961).

7. L. H. Roddis, *A Short History of Nautical Medicine* (New York: Hoeber, 1941), p. 106.

8. Dougal Robertson, *Survive the Savage Sea* (New York: Praeger, 1973), and Maurice Bailey and Maralyn Bailey, *Staying Alive* (New York: McKay, 1974).

9. Some authorities, such as Dr. Bernard Robin, have misrepresented the Robertsons' position, suggesting that they advocated using seawater. This is puzzling, since in both *Survive the Savage Sea* and *Sea Survival* (New York: Praeger, 1975), a second book by Robertson, it is clearly stated that seawater should not be given in this manner!

10. Robertson, *Survive the Savage Sea*, pp. 52-53.

11. Bernard Robin has collected 31 shipwreck stories in a fascinating book entitled *Survival at Sea* (Camden, Maine: International Marine Publishing, and London: Stanley Paul, 1981). The second part of the book is devoted to an analysis of a number of aspects of survival.

12. British Department of Trade, "Drinking of Sea Water by Castaways," Merchant Shipping Notice no. M.729, August 1975.

13. Lee and Lee, *Safety and Survival*, p. 152.

14. Robertson, *Survive the Savage Sea*, p. 244.

15. Surgeon Captain Walters's comments can be found in Bailey and Bailey, *Staying Alive*, pp. 187-191.

4

Sailor's Skin

*Mad dogs and Englishmen go out in
the midday sun;
The Japanese don't care to, the
Chinese wouldn't dare to;
Hindus and Argentines sleep firmly
from twelve to one.*

Noel Coward, *Mad Dogs and Englishmen*

S INCE THE 1970S, A quiet revolution has occurred that has radically altered our attitude toward the sun and its effect on our skin. Unabashed sun worship, only to achieve the darkest suntan in the shortest time, has given way to an increasing awareness of the long-term consequences of sun exposure—premature skin aging and an increased risk of skin cancer. Nowhere is this revolution more visible than in the cosmetics industry's marketing of sun lotions. Whereas the emphasis in the past was on quick tanning (which as we will see is not possible anyway), manufacturers now advertise their products' protective value as sun blockers or sunscreens.

This raised level of consciousness comes none too soon for sailors, who

71

have always been at risk to sustain solar (actinic) skin damage. In fact, the high prevalence of actinic damage among sailors prompted the term *sailor's skin* to describe the typical dry, wrinkled, inelastic, leathery skin of those who have spent years out in the midday sun. Unfortunately, these skin changes are irreversible, so prevention is absolutely essential. Fortunately, it is now possible to avoid actinic damage by partially or completely screening out the source of the damage—ultraviolet radiation.[1]

ULTRAVIOLET (UV) RADIATION

The sun continually emits a broad spectrum of radiation, ranging from gamma rays to radio-frequency waves. Fortunately for humans, only a tiny portion of this spectrum, the UV radiation, is injurious (Figure 4.1). The longer wavelengths, such as the visible and infrared, produce light and heat but have no adverse effect on the skin. The atmosphere with its protective layer of ozone filters out the shorter gamma, X, and some of the UV rays—all exceedingly dangerous to humans.

For convenience, UV radiation has been divided into three bands: UV-C (200 to 280 nanometers), UV-B (280 to 320 nanometers), and UV-A (320 to 400 nanometers). UV-C, although potentially dangerous, is of no concern to us since it is completely absorbed by the ozone layer and is not detectable at sea level. UV-B and UV-A do penetrate the atmosphere to varying degrees and are responsible for sunburning and suntanning, as well as actinic damage and skin cancer.

The effect of UV on the sailor's skin depends on two factors: (1) the cumulative dose of UV that the sailor receives and (2) the pigmentary defenses that the sailor can muster.

UV Exposure

First, let us examine what determines the amount of UV that actually reaches the sailor. This information is important, for the sailor must *anticipate* when he is likely to be exposed to significant UV. Only then can he take steps to protect himself. Once the skin is sunburned it is too late. He has already sustained radiation damage. If the immediate sunburn were the only concern, there would be no need for alarm. A sunburn, after all, heals. However, both actinic damage and skin cancer result from the cumulative dosage of UV radiation over a lifetime! Every episode of ex-

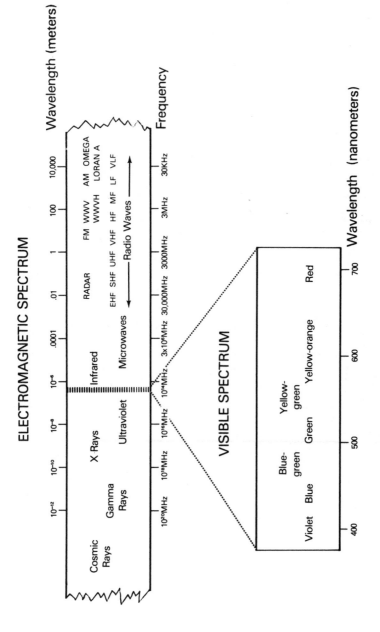

Figure 4.1. The electromagnetic radiation spectrum.

posure to the sun has, in a sense, left its radiational footprints in the sailor's epidermis.[2]

Unlike sunlight and infrared radiation, which can be seen and felt, UV radiation is entirely insensible. We can judge its presence only retrospectively by the degree of burn it leaves behind. Usually, UV traverses the atmosphere together with light and heat, which alert us to the danger. Sometimes, however, this warning system breaks down. Sailors are particularly vulnerable to a breakdown in the warning system since a moving boat generates a cooling breeze. It is easy in such circumstances to underestimate UV exposure. The warning system also breaks down on cloudy days when more UV penetrates the atmosphere than either light or heat.

How much UV penetrates to sea level depends primarily upon the particles present in the atmosphere. They filter out all radiation below 280 nanometers, including UV-C, as well as much of the UV-B and UV-A. The degree of obliquity with which the UV strikes the atmosphere also determines the amount of UV penetration. The greater the obliquity, the longer the course; and the longer the course, the greater the opportunity the UV has to be absorbed or scattered. The ozone (O_3) layer, located in the stratosphere 9 to 22 miles (15 to 35 kilometers) above the surface of the earth, plays a vital supporting role in the absorption of UV.

The most dangerous period for UV exposure is *midday* between the hours of 10 a.m. and 2 p.m. standard time (or, more precisely, local time). During these 4 hours, approximately 66 percent of the daily UV radiation reaches the surface of the earth; and between 9 a.m. and 3 p.m., over 80 percent. During the midday hours, the sun is highest in the sky, and the UV rays travel a more direct, less oblique course through the atmosphere.

Increased UV radiation in the *summer* and in *equatorial regions* has a similar explanation. The summer sun is higher in the sky (more nearly overhead) than is the winter sun. In equatorial regions, the sun is more directly overhead at midday than it is at higher latitudes. In addition, the ozone layer is not distributed uniformly around the earth. It tends to be thinner at the equator than at the poles. This alone increases the UV load by about 15 percent.

Probably the most neglected source of UV is the sky! The sky appears blue because the shorter blue wavelengths of light are more scattered than are the longer red and green wavelengths. After bouncing around the atmosphere, the blue rays are eventually reflected back to earth. Similarly, much of the UV reaches the earth after being scattered throughout the sky. (This makes sense since UV is immediately adjacent to the blue portion of the electromagnetic spectrum.). *This indirect "sky radiation" accounts for almost 50 percent of the total UV that reaches the earth on a clear day.* As a result, one can obtain a nasty sunburn even when standing in a shadow! The sailor invariably overlooks sky radiation, although it undoubtedly contributes to his above-average exposure. On the water, the expanse of open sky comprises a full 360 degrees—all of it radiating UV. The situation is obviously much different than in an urban setting where buildings and trees block out much of the sky radiation. In short, turning a back on the sun is not the answer.

The amount of UV radiated on a cloudy day is often underestimated as well. Because of its shorter wavelength, UV penetrates moderate cloud cover at a time when light and heat cannot. Up to 80 percent UV transmission can occur with complete cloud cover. Under exceptional circumstances (high, towering clouds), the amount of UV may actually be greater—due to increased backscatter—than that radiated from a cloudless sky.

Contrary to popular belief, water is a poor reflector of UV. At midday only about 5 to 10 percent is reflected from the surface. The percentage increases only slightly when the sun is lower in the sky. Although this benefits the sailor while he is sailing (otherwise the UV load would be even greater), when he takes to the water to swim or snorkel, he must consider that he will absorb UV while in the water. Such a situation can be extremely deceiving since the relative coolness of the water engenders a sense of security. When high UV radiation is anticipated, as in the Caribbean at midday, clothing and/or sunscreens are required while swimming or snorkeling. The sailor should beware of thinly woven materials such as nylon, which may allow 25 percent or more of UV transmission.

Finally, the best available evidence indicates that high temperature, high humidity, and high wind velocity all augment UV damage. Extra precaution should be taken in these conditions.

Sunburn

Sensitivity to UV varies considerably from individual to individual and depends on the amount of pigment, or *melanin,* in the superficial layers of the skin.[3] Melanin absorbs and scatters the UV, preventing its transmission to the deeper layers of the skin. In dark-complexioned individuals, melanin is present in the skin in large quantities even in the absence of sun exposure. In medium-complexioned individuals, little melanin is stored in the skin; but in response to UV, melanin is produced, a process referred to as tanning. In people with very fair skins, not only is there little or

TABLE 4.1
Skin Types

Type	Classification	Reaction to Sun Exposure
1	Very sensitive	Always burns, never tans
2	Sensitive	Always burns, minimally tans
3	Normal	Sometimes burns, always tans
4	Normal	Rarely burns, always tans
5	Insensitive	Never burns, always tans
6	Insensitive	Deeply pigmented (black)

no melanin stored in the skin, but the ability to produce it is either poor or absent. About 15 percent of people are entirely incapable of developing a suntan! These people are the most sensitive to the adverse effects of solar radiation.

Human skin has been divided into six basic types based on the amount of melanin normally stored in the skin and on the skin's ability to produce it (Table 4.1). *The amount of melanin naturally found in the skin (natural skin color) as well as the capacity to produce melanin (ability to tan) are genetically inherited traits, and nothing can be done to alter them. This applies to both the rate and the end result.* Quick tanning, therefore, is a myth, pure and simple. Tanning proceeds at its own pace for any given individual and depends primarily on the amount of UV received in a specific period of time.[4]

The first evidence of UV exposure is a very faint redness, or *erythema,* of the skin that develops during the exposure and disappears almost immediately. Unfortunately, a latent period of 2 to 4 hours follows before the erythema that we usually associate with sunburn appears. Because of this delay, the unwary sailor may develop a severe burn before he realizes that his exposure has been excessive. This erythema reaches its peak at about 24 hours and begins to subside after 72 hours. Depending on the severity, it may persist for up to 10 days.

If the exposure is mild, erythema is faintly visible at 24 hours. The amount of radiation that produces this minimal erythema is known as the *minimal erythema dose* (MED). This dose varies from individual to individual depending on skin type. The time it takes to absorb 1 MED also depends on the time of day, season, and latitude, as discussed earlier. For example, a medium-complexioned, untanned individual exposed to mid-

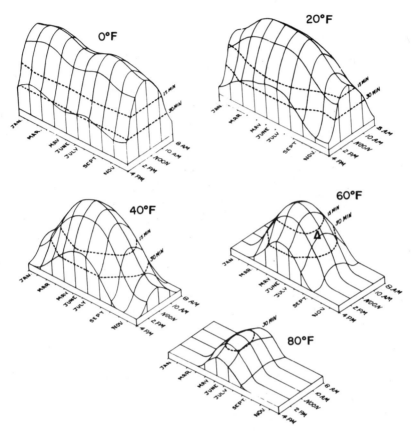

Figure 4.2. Minimal erythema dose (MED) in relation to latitude, season, and time of day. Reproduced, by permission, from F. Daniels, Jr., "Radiant Energy," in Environmental Physiology, *edited by N. B. Slonim (St. Louis: Mosby, 1974).*

day, midsummer sun at 41° north latitude (New York) receives 1 MED in about 15 minutes. In an area of higher UV intensity, such as Florida, the same individual may absorb 1 MED in only 10 minutes. The graphs in Figure 4.2 represent the time in which an average person receives 1 MED as a function of the time of day, season, and latitude. Extrapolated from actual measurements of UV, these graphs should be used as *rough* guides rather than reliable, safe indicators of sun exposure. The only accurate way for a sailor to know the time it will take for him to receive 1 MED in a particular region is by trial and error. Usually, he can estimate fairly accurately for his home port. For example, a medium-to-dark-complexioned sailor may know that he normally requires 30 minutes of midday, midsummer, Chesapeake sun to provoke a faint erythema 24 hours after his first exposure of the season.

Even though this estimated time to receive 1 MED is rough, it is important. What happens when it is exceeded? If exposure is extended so that the skin absorbs 2.5 MED, the result is a vivid and mildly painful erythema. A 5 MED sunburn is not only red but decidedly painful, whereas a 10 MED exposure produces a severe sunburn with subsequent blistering. Exposures of this degree are usually followed within 4 to 7 days by peeling of the epidermal layer. The area of peeling exposes pink, unprotected, supersensitive skin, which may be so damaged that it is not capable of producing any melanin for the next few months!

UV-B is the major culprit. It produces 90 percent of the sunburn damage, whereas UV-A is only responsible for about 10 percent. (Actually, UV-B is 1,000 times as burning as UV-A, but more UV-A penetrates to sea level.) The most dangerous wavelength is 305 nanometers, right in the middle of the UV-B band. Because of this, most of the earlier sunscreens were directed primarily or exclusively toward eliminating UV-B wavelengths. This approach is no longer acceptable. First, very sensitive skins—especially type 1—can still burn from pure UV-A. Second, it is unclear how much actinic damage and/or skin cancer is due to UV-B, how much to UV-A, or how much to a combination of the two. Third, a number of widely used medications sensitize the skin to UV radiation, a process called *photosensitivity*. Table 4.2 lists the most common photosensitizing drugs. Most of the photosensitivity reactions are due to UV-A, not UV-B. It is important that the sailor select a sunscreen directed against both UV-A and UV-B (see discussion later in the chapter).

Tanning

Both sunburn and suntan result from UV that has been transmitted through the layers of the skin. But whereas sunburn causes only damage (both immediate and cumulative), tanning serves a useful purpose. A well-developed tan provides some protection from future UV radiation. Unfortunately, to obtain a tan, a person must first suffer at least a mild burn. For those who are able to tan, the goal should always be to minimize this unavoidable burn.

Most people envisage the tanning process as a simple photochemical reaction; sunlight strikes the skin and somehow produces darkening of skin pigment. Actually, the process is slightly more complex and far more interesting.

TABLE 4.2
Drugs That May Produce Photosensitivity

1. *Phenothiazines.* These drugs are used primarily as major tranquilizers although promethazine (Phenergan) is primarily used to treat nausea and is very effective for motion sickness.
  • examples include chlorpromazine (Thorazine), thioridazine (Mellaril), trifluoperazine (Stelazine), promethazine (Phenergan); see also Table 3.2
2. *Tetracyclines.* Any of the drugs in the tetracycline group may cause photosensitivity, but the most common agent is demeclocycline.
  • examples include demeclocycline (Declomycin), oxytetracycline (Oxytetracycline, Terramycin), doxycycline (Vibramycin), tetracycline (Achromycin, Sumycin)
3. *Nalidixic Acid (NegGram).* This drug is used to treat urinary tract infections. Skin sensitivity may continue for up to 2 months after the drug has been discontinued.
4. *Sulfa Drugs.* Any of the sulfa drugs may on occasion produce photosensitivity; the most common offender is sulfanilamide, which is not used frequently at the present time.
5. *Diuretics (Antihypertension).*
  • examples include chlorothiazide (Diuril), hydrochlorothiazide (Hydrodiuril), furosemide (Lasix)
6. *Miscellaneous.* Oral contraceptives, amantadine (Symmetrel), diphenhydramine (Benedryl), and griseofulvin have *occasionally* produced photosensitivity.
7. Various cosmetics applied to the skin and even on occasion sunscreens themselves may produce photosensitivity.

The skin is composed of two parts, the epidermis and the dermis (see Figure 3.1). Tanning is confined exclusively to the epidermis. At the base of the epidermis are specialized cells called *melanocytes,* which manufacture melanin in response to UV (Figure 4.3). Of course, if the melanin is to diminish UV transmission through the skin, it must somehow be transferred to the surface. Nature accomplishes this by an ingenious method. The melanin is packaged into disklike structures called *melanosomes.* These melanosomes are then distributed to the other cells of the epidermis called *keratinocytes,* via processes known as dendrites because of their resemblance to nerve cell terminals.[5] In the human epidermis, each melanocyte is associated with about 36 keratinocytes. Together the melanocyte and its 36 keratinocytes constitute the *epidermal melanin unit.* Human skin contains a very large number of these units—1,000 to 2,000 per square millimeter.

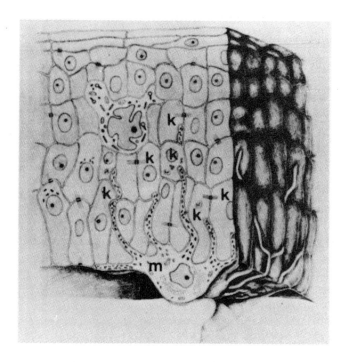

Figure 4.3. *The epidermal melanin unit, illustrating a melanocyte* (m) *and some of its associated keratinocytes* (k). *Reproduced, by permission, from W. C. Quevedo, Jr., "The control of color in mammals,"* American Zoology, *vol. 9 (1969).*

Once the melanosome is transferred to the keratinocyte, it remains within and travels with the keratinocyte to the skin surface during the normal process of skin regeneration. When the keratinocyte reaches the surface, it and the melanin within it are shed.

When sufficient UV penetrates the skin, two distinct phenomena occur. Under the influence of UV-A there is *immediate pigment darkening,* which is a photochemical response of the melanin already present in the skin. Immediate pigment darkening lasts only a few hours, although faint traces may persist for 1 to 2 days. Under the influence of UV-B primarily, the skin undergoes both burning (erythema) and true tanning. Exactly how UV-B excites the melanocyte to produce the melanosomes remains a mystery. One theory is that the initial step involves a small amount of UV-B–induced radiation damage to the DNA or RNA within the melanocyte.

The process of true tanning requires time: time for the production of the melanosomes, time for the transfer of the melanosomes to the keratinocytes, and time for the keratinocytes to ascend to the skin surface. This explains the 3- to 6-day latent period for true tanning; that is, for the first 3 to 6 days, the only noticeable change in the color of the skin is due to erythema, not tanning! And if during this period the skin is burned severely enough to produce peeling, the entire process must begin anew.

SUN PROTECTION

With misleading advertising, the cosmetics industry has fostered the popular misconception that creams and lotions can actually promote tanning (hence the term *suntan lotions*). This is patently false. These substances when applied to the skin permit—but do not promote—tanning in proportion to the amount of UV that is allowed to reach the skin. We must dispense with both the term and the concept of the suntan and evaluate these substances as sunscreens.

All sunscreens protect the skin by either absorbing or reflecting UV. Although there is considerable interest in the development of an oral sunscreen, to date all sunscreen agents must be applied directly to the skin.[6]

In choosing a sunscreen, several factors should be taken into consideration: (1) the individual's skin type (Table 4.1); (2) the degree of protection provided—known as the sun protection factor (SPF); (3) the absorption spectrum—UV-B, UV-A, or both; (4) the cost, which varies widely; and (5) the particular disadvantages of specific preparations.

Individual sensitivity determines not only a person's choice of a particular sunscreen but his entire attitude toward the sun! Sailors with type 1 and probably type 2 skin should forget about tanning and concentrate entirely on protection. These sailors should choose sunscreen agents with the highest SPF and the broadest spectrum across both UV-B and UV-A. They should wear broad-rimmed hats and employ other forms of physical protection whenever possible. Close-weave garments provide almost complete protection. The helmsman, during the midday period, might consider a pair of light gloves. Because of man's upright posture, certain areas receive more than average UV and require above-average protection: the nose, the tops of the ears, the lower lip, the upper back, and the area where the chest meets the neck. Also, don't forget the back of the neck, behind the knees, and insteps!

At the other extreme, individuals with types 5 and 6 skin require little protection. Nonetheless, they should not become complacent. There is no reason to court later skin damage and skin cancer (both of which are *less* likely to occur with these skin types) when protection is readily available. It certainly seems prudent to seek protection at least for periods of high UV exposure.

Skin types 3 and 4 present the greatest challenge. These people do have something to gain from *controlled* UV exposure (the protection of a well-developed tan) as well as something to lose (actinic damage and cancer).

In order to facilitate the selection of an appropriate sunscreen, the U.S. Food and Drug Administration has mandated that each sunscreen be identified by its SPF. SPF is a measure of the effectiveness of the sunscreen, regardless of the specific active ingredient, or, simply stated, a ratio of the MED with and without the sunscreen:

$$\text{SPF} = \frac{\text{MED with sunscreen}}{\text{MED without sunscreen}}$$

For example, let us return to the sailor who usually requires 30 minutes of midday, midsummer Chesapeake sun to receive 1 MED. His particular MED time for these conditions would be 30 minutes. If he applied a sunscreen with an SPF of eight, it would now take 240 minutes (4 hours) of exposure to produce his minimal erythema (1 MED). The sunscreen has increased by 8 times the amount of time the sailor can remain in the sun and still only receive 1 MED. If, however, we take the same sailor and expose him to a midday equatorial sun, his MED time might drop to only 10 minutes. In this case a sunscreen preparation with an SPF of 8 would allow him to receive 1 MED in only 80 minutes. If he were exposed to 4 hours of midday sun, he would end up with 3 MED (240 minutes in the sun ÷ 80 minutes per MED) and a vivid erythema.

Once the sailor estimates the time it takes to develop 1 MED and the probable length of his exposure, he can choose a sunscreen with an appropriate SPF. Near the equator, for example, an SPF of 15 would allow an average sailor to stay out in the midday sun for 150 minutes before developing 1 MED. If he were planning to stay out for all 4 peak hours (10 a.m. to 2 p.m.), he would expect to receive about 1.6 MED (240 minutes ÷ 150 minutes per MED). Obviously, these calculations are only rough approximations. But at least the sailor has some idea of the amount of protection he is receiving. SPF values from less than 4 to 15 and above are available, but since only a few strengths are likely to be on board at any one time, close approximations are all that can be expected. Needless to say, the sailor has nothing to lose by erring on the side of overprotection.

It turns out that the fastest (but not necessarily the safest) *way to achieve a tan is to receive 2 MED per day.* Even at this rate, it still takes about 14 days to develop a consummate tan. Increasing the MED does not hasten the process. It increases only the risk of damage and may produce enough of a burn to promote peeling. Sailors who are chronically exposed to UV should not be interested in achieving the fastest tan anyway. Their major concern should be to reduce the amount of damage. Consequently, they should limit exposure to less than 2 MED per day if possible.

It is worth noting that as the sailor begins to tan, he needs to revise his estimate of his MED time; that is, after the 3- to 6-day latent period, the newly developed tan begins to offer "natural" protection. At this point the sailor has two choices if he wishes to keep his MED constant, say, at 2. He can either decrease the SPF of his sunscreen or he can increase his exposure time. Since the mild erythema that is the hallmark of 1 MED is difficult to discern in the presence of a tan, the revised estimate must be pure guesswork.

Sunscreens

The active ingredient in most sunscreens falls into one of three categories: (1) para-aminobenzoic acid (PABA) or one of its derivatives, (2) non-PABA chemical sunscreens, or (3) physical sunscreens.

PABA and its derivatives are extremely popular.[7] There are, however, two disadvantages. First, they tend to stain lightly colored fabrics and occasionally they may even damage a fiberglass finish. Second, PABA and its derivatives are only effective against UV-B; they allow full transmission of UV-A. People who are very sensitive or who are taking any of the medications listed in Table 4.2 should avoid *pure* PABA preparations. Because of these drawbacks, other non-PABA sunscreens have been developed. The major chemical groups include the benzophenones, the salicylates, the cinnamates, and the acrilonitriles. The benzophenones (oxybenzone and dioxybenzone) are unique among the chemical sunscreens in that they are effective against UV-A. Most of the newer chemical sunscreens on the market (except for the weakest) have combined PABA or one of its derivatives with a benzophenone to block both UV-B and UV-A (see Table 4.3).

The physical sunscreens were the first to be developed. They include such ingredients as zinc oxide, titanium dioxide, kaolin, talc, and iron oxide. These agents are for the most part opaque, which means that they absorb light as well as UV-B and UV-A. Since they are usually available only as thick concoctions, not as lotions or creams, they are not practical

TABLE 4.3
Examples of U.S. Sunscreen Preparations

	SPF	Active Ingredients
Presun	4	4% octyl dimethyl PABA (Padimate 0)
Presun	8	5% PABA
Presun	15	5% PABA, 5% Padimate 0, 3% oxybenzone
Sundown	6	5.3% Padimate 0, 1.75% oxybenzone
Sundown	8	7% Padimate 0, 2% oxybenzone, 5% octyl salicylate
Sundown	15	7% Padimate 0, 4% oxybenzone, 5% octyl salicylate
Shade	6	8% homosalate, 3% oxybenzone
Super Shade	15	7% Padimate 0, 3% oxybenzone
Bain de Soleil	8	3.5% Padimate 0, 0.6% oxybenzone
Bain de Soleil	15	7% Padimate 0, 2.5% oxybenzone, 0.5% dioxybenzone

for protecting large areas of the body as are the chemical sunscreens. Their primary usefulness is in protecting small sensitive areas such as the cheeks, nose, lips, ears, and bald spots. When applied liberally, these agents virtually exclude any UV from reaching the skin.

There are a number of practical tips for the use of any of the sunscreens, especially the chemical agents:

1. Apply all preparations to clean, dry skin. PABA, for example, is not water soluble. If it is applied to wet skin, it precipitates, forming tiny crystals that are completely ineffective.

2. All preparations, especially those that contain PABA, should be applied at least 1 hour prior to exposure. This measure seems to afford longer protection and also increases the resistance to erosion by sweating or swimming. The interval of time may be necessary for the PABA to bind to the outer layers of the skin.

3. Repeated applications are still necessary after swimming or exercise.

4. In addition to those "sensitive" spots, beware of overlooking certain areas that are usually not associated with sunburning (see earlier discussion).

SUNBURN TREATMENT

On occasions when a sailor or one of his crew members miscalculates his exposure, certain steps can be taken to treat sunburn. Cool water compresses or immersion may offer symptomatic relief and, if given early enough, reduce blistering.

For limited areas of severe burn (5 to 10 MED), steroid cream such as hydrocortisone may relieve the pain and reduce the inflammation. Hydrocortisone cream in strengths up to 0.5 percent is now available over the counter. Higher concentrations still require a physician's prescription. Local anesthetics such as any of the *caine* ointments—benzocaine (Solarcaine) or dibucaine (Nupercainal)—are also of temporary benefit. Aspirin or acetaminophen (Tylenol) in the usual dosage is also effective in relieving the pain.

An extensive, severe burn with blistering demands a more aggressive approach. A short course of high-dose oral steroids such as prednisone is sometimes helpful. Oral steroids are not without hazards, however, and the sailor using them should be under the care of a physician.

OTHER SKIN DISORDERS

Prickly Heat (Heat Rash)

Prickly heat, officially known as miliaria, might appear to be too trivial for the sailor's consideration, but it is not. Although minor individual attacks are inconsequential, repeated or extensive episodes can leave the sailor in jeopardy.

Prickly heat occurs when it is hot and humid, and when sweating has been prolonged and copious. The skin lesions, *which always appear at the sweat pores,* may be crystal clear or opaque like gooseflesh, but most commonly they resemble tiny blood blisters. They may sting, itch, or burn. Portions of the skin that are covered are most vulnerable, especially when the clothing creates friction. The palms and soles are never involved, the face only rarely.

The rash erupts whenever the free flow of sweat is impeded. For reasons not entirely clear, keratin from the outermost layer of the epidermis plugs the sweat duct, blocking further sweat flow to the surface (Figure 3.1). In the absence of sweat, the eruption fades in a couple of days. If sweating begins, the rash promptly recurs, and each recurrence tends to involve more sweat glands.

The major concern for the sailor is that extensive prickly heat predisposes to heatstroke (see Chapter 3). But even in the absence of heatstroke, repeated episodes impair sweating efficiency and reduce exercise tolerance.

Prickly heat can be prevented. Clothing should be loose and well ventilated. A high salt intake can occasionally precipitate and sometimes aggravate it. The best preventive is to avoid the heat. Between 4 and 6 hours per day in a cool environment appears to be sufficient to prevent the disorder.

Seawater Boils

Seawater boils result from a bacterial infection of the hair follicles (Figure 4.3). The bacteria *(Staphylococcus)* are normally harmless inhabitants of the skin. However, when exposed to constant wetness, which is often unavoidable at sea, these bacteria grow, resulting in infection. Anything that irritates the skin, such as the friction of clothing, hastens the process.

Bob Griffith discusses the problem the cruising sailor faces in *Blue Water*. He refers to the condition as helmsman's rear end, since that is the boils' most common location:

> This is the term we coined for the small sea boils or pustules located in the gluteal region that so commonly afflict small-boat sailors at sea. It is best prevented and best treated by keeping dry, and to this end I advise everyone not to wear underpants. While outer pants wet with saltwater dry in the air, underwear stays damp and the skin remains soft and irritated by salt and the pressure of sitting. Helmsman's Rear End results when bacteria infect the hair follicles or pores of the skin. In warm weather, when one isn't always careful about remaining dry on watch or working on the foredeck, Helmsman's Rear End sometimes is so bad that we have a daily clinic. The pustules are opened, drained, and dotted with dilute (1 to 100) formalin, tincture of iodine or other antiseptic, which is followed by a 20-minute sun treatment of the affected area.
>
> Saltwater boils on wrists and calves where cuffs and boots rub are a related affliction but worse because they inhibit a sailor's movements and are likely to be reopened in the course of deck work. They yield to essentially the same treatment, but may require oral antibiotics. And they must be protected from abrasion from the cuff or boot that caused them.[8]

Swimmer's Itch

Swimmer's itch (also known as clam-digger's itch and swamp itch) is caused by the infestation of the skin with tiny parasites, the flukes. Of the numerous species of flukes, some are capable of parasitizing man, causing *schistosomiasis,* a serious disease prevalent in many parts of the world. These species are exclusively freshwater inhabitants, and for this reason caution is necessary when swimming in unfamiliar lakes, ponds, and streams (see "Miscellaneous Health Hints," Chapter 7).

The species that cause swimmer's itch are not capable of causing schistosomiasis, only a dermatitis. These species are widely distributed throughout the freshwater areas of the world as well as some brackish and coastal waters (including the Atlantic seaboard, the Gulf coast, California, and Hawaii).

The initial exposure to the parasites usually produces a mild prickling and itching sensation after a person emerges from the water. As the film of water evaporates, the parasites penetrate the skin. Small skin lesions follow but usually disappear in a few days in nonsensitized people. In a person sensitized by a previous exposure, however, the reaction is often worse and may persist for 1 to 2 weeks.

Usually the skin lesions predominate on exposed areas of the body, less frequently on areas that clothing or a bathing suit covers. Treatment usually consists of medication to relieve the itching. There is evidence that drying the skin thoroughly, *immediately after exposure,* may prevent the penetration of many of the organisms.

NOTES

1. The term *ultraviolet light* is frequently used, although, strictly speaking, *light* refers only to radiation with a wavelength between 400 and 760 nanometers, making it visible to the human eye. (A nanometer is a billionth of a meter.)

2. The situation is analogous to that of X-ray exposure. The precise manner in which the X-rays are received is usually less important than the cumulative dosage over a lifetime. A lifetime of minor "insults" may be just as injurious as a lesser number of severe exposures.

3. A few individuals are *unusually* sensitive to UV. They may experience welts, blisters, or skin lesions that look somewhat like juvenile acne. Since most of these conditions begin in childhood or adolescence, the sensitive individuals invariably are aware of their condition.

4. There are lotions available that chemically react with the skin to produce an orange-brown hue. Although they are referred to as tanning lotions, they bear no relation to the natural tanning process. Also, an artificial carotenoid dye may soon be marketed in the United States as a "tanning pill." This dye stains the subcutaneous fat a yellowish-brown color, producing a tanned appearance. These cosmetic innovations can be dangerous if the resemblance to natural tanning leads to complacency. (N.B.: Artificial skin coloring by cosmetics of any type offers no protection whatsoever against solar radiation!)

5. The resemblance between the tanning process and central nervous system activity is by no means fortuitous. During early human development, the melanocytes (or, more properly, their precursors the melanoblasts) migrated to the skin from early central nervous system tissue. In other words, melanocytes are first cousins to the nerve cells in the brain. Many of the nutrients and enzymes are

exactly the same. A prominent example is dopa. Dopa plays an important role in transmitting nerve impulses in the brain, and its absence in a specific region of the brain produces Parkinson's disease. It turns out that dopa is also the major ingredient in the production of melanin.

6. Para-aminobenzoic acid (PABA), an active ingredient in many sunscreen preparations, is available in oral form. It is sold as a nutritional supplement in health-food stores. Sailors should be advised that oral PABA provides no sunscreen protection whatsoever!

7. Glyceryl PABA, octydimethyl PABA (Padimate O), and iso-amyl-para-N,N-dimethyl-aminobenzoate (Padimate A) represent three PABA derivatives that are frequently found in various sunscreens. As a general rule, never purchase a sunscreen unless its active ingredients are listed. You should be able to recognize either a PABA or a non-PABA ingredient (or both) among the active ingredients. If not, choose again!

8. Bob Griffith with Nancy Griffith, *Blue Water* (Boston: Sail Books, 1979), pp. 184-185.

5

Sailing Nutrition

*Serve God daily, love one another,
and preserve your victuals.*

Sir John Hawkins, 1562 (advice to
his crew prior to embarkation)

NOWADAYS IT SEEMS THAT sailors are interested mostly in the
gastronomic aspects of food. New recipes for the shipboard preparation of old favorites, as well as recommendations for the compleat nautical
wine list, are the order of the day. Although there is nothing wrong with
epicurism (except perhaps when coupled with decadence!), the nautical
community's neglect of nutrition is a pity. Sailors of every stripe need
to know at least *something* about the food they eat. It is especially rele-
vant today, when the health food industry continually barrages us with
claims concerning such-and-such a vitamin or food supplement.

Nutrition is also part of our nautical heritage. In the past, food and
drink were of vital concern in the planning of ocean voyages. Inadequate

storage, food spoilage, and vitamin deficiencies (either unrecognized or ignored) were ever-present problems. The early explorers of the New World, for example, were limited by the amount of food they could carry. A voyage to the West Indies was just about the longest and farthest possible, and several times food gave out on unduly prolonged return voyages. No mariner prior to Sir Francis Drake managed to feed his crew properly on any voyage into the Southern Hemisphere, especially those that reached the Pacific Ocean. As Captain Morison points out,

> There simply was not room enough, or storage tight enough, to preserve basic foodstuffs, such as wine, hard bread, flour, and salt meat, for so long a time. Hence the resort to penguin meat, seal, and other loathsome substitutes; and occasionally to the desperate eating of rats and chewing leather chafing-gear. Drake's men made out comparatively well, only because he stripped every prize ship of all desirable food stores, gear, and weapons. There is not one of these southern voyages on which the modern blue-water yachtsman, used to refrigeration and canned goods, would have been happy.[1]

As longer voyages became routine during the 17th and 18th centuries, the problem of storage was replaced by that of food spoilage and infestation. The daily allowance for each man in the Royal Navy during this period was

Biscuit	1 lb daily
Salt beef	2 lb twice weekly
Salt pork	1 lb twice weekly
Dried fish	2 oz thrice weekly
Oatmeal	1/2 pt thrice weekly
Butter	2 oz thrice weekly
Cheese	4 oz thrice weekly
Peas	8 oz four times weekly
Beer	1 gal daily

The caloric value of this ration (if we include the beer at about 130 calories per pint) is roughly 3,800 calories. The quantity of food was not at fault however. The amount was "greater than to satisfy an ordinary eater." Rather, the principal objection lay in the quality. This ration contained no fresh foodstuffs and, apart from traces in the beer, was totally lacking in vitamin C. As Captain Roddis remarks, "The pickling process destroyed much of the flavor and palatability of the beef and pork and unfavorably affected their nutrient value. Many stories are told of the beef. It was said that when old and allowed to dry, it could be carved into small boxes or figures which, if shellacked, had much the appearance and the consistency of mahogany."[2]

The staple of the sailor's diet was his sea bread, or biscuit, what we know today as hard bread, or hardtack. "It was often as hard as flint and all too frequently infested with weevils. Knocking the bread against the edge of the mess table in order to remove the weevils was a regular practice and the noise made by the procedure was as regular a sound at meal time as the rattle of mess gear."[3]

The amount of beer may seem surprising, but in part it compensated for the lack of fresh water aboard ship. The quality was poor, and eventually rum, generally known as grog, was issued instead.[4]

THE SAILOR'S DIET

Obviously, things have come a long way. It is now recognized that a sailor's diet should supply all of the required nutrients for energy, maintenance and repair of body tissue, and growth. The simple "four-food-group" system is still the best scheme for menu planning (Table 5.1). Menus formulated from these guidelines should include 12 servings for adults, selected from the four groups. Growing children and adolescents require increased servings from the milk group. The four-food-group system has enough latitude to be practical at sea, no matter how limited the space for provisions. A reasonably balanced diet contains approximately 55 to 58 percent of the calories in the form of carbohydrates, no more than 30 percent as fat, and about 12 to 15 percent in the form of protein.[5]

Protein

There is nothing magical about protein. It is composed of various combinations of 20 amino acid "building blocks." The way in which the different amino acids are put together determines the structure and function of the particular protein. The adult body cannot synthesize eight of the amino acids, which therefore must be provided in the diet. These are referred to as the essential amino acids. Infants cannot synthesize an additional amino acid. The proportion of amino acids in a protein determines its nutritional value. *Complete protein* contains all of the essential amino acids in approximately the correct ratio. All of the building blocks are supplied at the same time and are available for the construction of any protein the body needs. *Incomplete protein* either lacks one or more

TABLE 5.1
The Four-Food-Group Plan

	Examples	Recommended daily servings		
		Adults	Children	Adolescents
1. Milk group	Milk, cheese, ice cream, sour cream, yogurt.	2	3	4
2. Meat and high-protein group	Meat, fish, shellfish, poultry, eggs. Because of high-protein value, dried beans, peas, nuts, and peanut butter can be used as alternatives.	2	2	2
3. Vegetable and fruit group	Dark green and deep yellow, rich in vitamin A; dark green and citrus fruits, rich in vitamin C.	4	4	4
4. Bread and cereal group	Enriched or fortified breads, cereals, flour, baked goods, or whole-grain products.	4	4	4

The following amounts each constitute one serving: 3.5 oz (100 grams) of meat or fish; 1 cup (8 oz) of milk or 1 oz of cheese; ½ cup of fruit or vegetables or ½ cup of juice; 1 slice of bread, 1 cup ready-to-eat cereal, or ½ cup of cooked cereal.

If large quantities of milk and milk products are consumed, fortified skim milk should be substituted to reduce the amount of saturated fat in the diet. Fish and chicken have significantly less saturated fat than other sources of protein.

of the essential amino acids or comprises them in an unusual ratio. However, combining a variety of incomplete sources, such as fruits, vegetables, and grains, accomplishes virtually the same result. The strengths and weaknesses of one protein complement those of the other, a concept known as *protein complementarity*. In this way, a vegetarian diet need not be inferior in protein quality to a diet that contains animal products.

By and large, animal protein is more complete than plant protein. The most complete sources are eggs, fish, beef, poultry, milk, and cheese. The following have a high amino acid content although they are incomplete: nuts, seeds (such as sunflower or sesame), lentils, peanut butter, beans, and peas.

Since protein is the major constituent of muscle, there must be protein in the diet to increase muscle mass. But, consuming huge amounts of protein does not augment muscle mass. *Only muscle work increases muscle mass.* Since the typical Western diet contains more than twice the amount of protein necessary and since active sailors frequently consume considerable quantities of food, their diet invariably contains two to three times the amount of protein needed to increase muscle mass. *All additional protein in the diet is simply broken down and used as fuel or stored as fat.* There is absolutely no evidence that protein supplementation in the form of tablets or liquids benefits either health or athletic performance!

Carbohydrates

The main function of carbohydrates is to provide energy. Carbohydrates that the body does not use immediately are stored in the liver and muscle as *glycogen,* which consists of hundreds and thousands of glucose sugar molecules that are linked together. Once the capacity for glycogen storage is reached, the remainder is stored as fat.

During exercise, glycogen, especially that stored in the particular muscles being exercised, breaks down, supplying a significant amount of fuel for the muscles. (The rest of the energy is supplied by the breakdown of fat into fatty acids, which are then burned as fuel.) Fatigue occurs if the glycogen in these muscles becomes depleted.

Athletes who are involved in endurance events (runners or bicyclists, for example) have discovered that by modifying their carbohydrate intake prior to an athletic event, they can increase the amount of glycogen in their muscles and improve their performance. This has been confirmed experimentally. Subjects were divided into three groups and given three different diets. The first group had a normal caloric intake, but most of the calories were in the form of fat. Group two was provided with the recommended percentages of fat, carbohydrate, and protein. The third group was given over 80 percent of their calories in the form of carbohydrate. The glycogen concentration in the leg muscles of these subjects averaged 0.6, 1.75, and 3.75 grams per 100 grams of muscle, respectively. The high carbohydrate group had significantly more glycogen in their muscles, and their endurance capacity was also markedly improved!

The technique of "carbohydrate loading," or "glycogen supercompensation," consists of two phases. In the initial phase, exhaustive exercise and a low carbohydrate intake for 3 to 4 days deplete the muscles of glycogen. Phase two consists of reduced activity and high carbohydrate intake for the 3 to 4 days right before competition. This regimen can increase glycogen stores *in those muscles that are exercised* by well over 100 percent. For most competitive sailors who perform primarily brief, nonendurance tasks, carbohydrate loading is usually not necessary. For endurance events, a *modified* loading is more practical than the two-phase technique. Instead of restricting carbohydrates early in the week and restricting activity later in the week, the athlete continues his intense training for the entire week prior to competition, increasing his carbohydrate intake by 1,000 to 1,500 calories (above normal caloric intake), for 3 to 4 days before the event. This increase will produce a glycogen concentration in the exercised muscles about 75 percent as high as the full carbohydrate-loading regimen. Remember, carbohydrate loading is to be used only prior to selected events. It is not intended as a routine diet.[6]

Carbohydrates come in two basic types, *simple* and *complex.* The simple carbohydrates include all of the sugars, such as glucose, fructose, sucrose, and lactose. There are two kinds of complex carbohydrates: starch and cellulose. It really doesn't matter how the racing sailor gets his carbohydrate, although the starches are generally more nutritious than the simple sugars. Everyone is familiar with the starches, but few people appreciate the importance of cellulose, especially for the cruising sailor. Cellulose is found in the fibrous part of plants and is present in the leaves, stems, seeds, roots, and the covering of fruit. Because cellulose is resistant to human digestive enzymes, it provides the food residue with "bulk" or "fiber," which aids in bowel movement. Cellulose is especially important for individuals who routinely become constipated at sea. One explanation for sea constipation is that sailors frequently become slightly dehydrated. Fluid intake is often less than on land and, if the weather is warm, a significant amount of water may be lost via sweating (see Chapter 3). In order to preserve body water, extra water is reabsorbed from the food residue, and this in turn produces constipation. Cellulose fiber, since it is hydrophilic, tends to counteract this action, promoting a more normal bowel movement. The commonly used bulk laxatives work in this fashion. Many utilize psyllium seed as a source of cellulose (e.g., Metamucil). If the sailor tends toward constipation, he should provide for either dietary or supplementary fiber in his diet.

Fats

Fats are not of great concern to the sailor. Of all the dietary fats, only one, linoleic acid, must be consumed; the body synthesizes the others. Linoleic acid is present in butter, cooking oils, and salad oils so that sufficient intake is difficult to avoid. As a sound general dietary rule, saturated fat (primarily from animal sources) should make up less than 33 percent of the total fat consumption.

Vitamins

Vitamins are the most misunderstood of all of the food substances. They neither supply energy to the body nor contribute to its mass. What they do is play a crucial role as catalysts in many of the body's metabolic reactions. As catalysts, vitamins are needed only in small quantities. They are used up very slowly, so their daily requirements are small.[7]

There are 14 vitamins: 10 water soluble (B_1, B_2, B_6, B_{12}, pantothenic acid, niacin, biotin, choline, folic acid, and vitamin C) and 4 fat soluble (A, D, E, K).

Since the fat-soluble vitamins are stored in the fatty tissues of the body, they need not be taken every day. In fact, it takes years for symptoms of a fat-soluble-vitamin deficiency to occur. Excessive intake, however, has risks. Large doses of vitamins A and D taken regularly eventually produce serious toxic effects. Although a true "overdose" of vitamins E and K is rare, intake above recommended levels offers no particular benefit.

The water-soluble vitamins—the B-complex and C—are not stored as extensively. Unlike the fat-soluble vitamins, excessive intake does not produce continued accumulation. Once the body's stores are replete, whatever is left over is excreted in the urine.

Athletes, because they have a higher total calorie intake, have a slightly higher requirement for three of the B-complex vitamins—thiamine (B_1), riboflavin (B_2), and niacin. Nevertheless, vitamin supplementation is not necessary since a varied diet contains an abundance of B-complex vitamins.

Experiments have demonstrated that on a diet that contains no vitamin C whatsoever, it takes 4 to 6 months to deplete the body's stores. For this reason, scurvy (a vitamin-C deficiency) did not become a nautical health problem until the Age of Exploration, when extended voyages were attempted. The saddest part of the scurvy story is that it need not have occurred!

As early as 1593, during a voyage to the South Pacific, Sir Richard Hawkins recommended the following treatment for scurvy: "That which I have seen most fruitfull for this sicknesse, is sower [sour] oranges and lemmons."[8] Better yet, only 7 years later, Captain James Lancaster unintentionally performed a *controlled study* of lemon juice as a preventive for scurvy. His fleet of four ships departed on April 2, 1601, and scurvy began to appear in three of the ships by August 1 (4 months after sailing). By the time of arrival, September 9, the three ships were so devastated by scurvy that the men of Lancaster's ship had to assist the rest of the fleet into the harbor. "And the reason why the General's [Lancaster's] men stood better in health than the men of other ships was this:—he brought to sea with him certaine bottles of the juice of limons, which he gave to each one as long as it would last, three spoonfuls every morning, fasting, not suffering them to eat anything after it till noone."[9]

Incredibly, the naval authorities ignored these discoveries, and scurvy continued to decimate the ranks of seamen. The account of Admiral George A. Anson's round-the-world voyage in the *Centurion* is gruesome testimony. In 1740 he embarked with six ships and 1,955 men in all. Four years later the flagship alone returned; 1,051 sailors died, mostly of scurvy!

Losses of this magnitude encouraged the Scottish naval surgeon James Lind to seek a cure. Aware of the earlier work, he performed his now-classic experiment in 1747 aboard the *Salisbury,* studying the effects of several types of treatment—including one composed of "two oranges and one lemon given every day"—on sailors with the typical signs of scurvy—"putrid gums, the spots and lassitude, with weakness of their knees." The curative power of these citrus fruits was clear, although with typical bureaucratic inertia, it was another 48 years before the Admiralty prescribed lemon juice for all British sailors. What finally persuaded the Admiralty was the experience of Captain James Cook. Less than 30 years after Anson's voyage, Cook made his first voyage of a little over 3 years and lost but one man from disease, probably tuberculosis! On board Cook pursued a slightly different tack. He relied heavily on malt and sauerkraut as preventives. For actual cases of scurvy he used orange and lemon juice, the limited supply of which the surgeon kept. Cook also sent men ashore at every opportunity to procure local fresh vegetables. In order to persuade his men to eat these exotic foods, he insisted that his officers eat them with tremendous gusto in front of the men. This ingenious strategy was so effective that rationing was sometimes necessary. Cook was the first commander to demonstrate conclusively that long ocean voyages did not necessarily result in scurvy or other health problems, an achievement in which he took pride.

Undoubtedly the scurvy story should end there, but there is one additional twist. For years, the victualing commissioners obtained their lemon juice from Sicily. However, in the 19th century it seemed feasible to replace the lemon with the lime, which was in plentiful supply in the West Indies. Since the juice of the lime was supposedly as good as that of the lemon, it was made the official antiscurvy treatment for the Royal Navy in 1860 (hence the term *limey*). Unfortunately, no one realized that preserved lime juice, unlike preserved lemon juice, contains little or no vitamin C. Outbreaks of scurvy reappeared until 1918, when it was proven conclusively with guinea pigs that lime juice had no antiscorbutic effect! The British navy estimates that during the worst years of the scurvy, between 1600 and 1800, nearly 5,000 lives were lost each year. That means that nearly 1,000,000 men died of an easily preventable disease—largely due to official indifference and stupidity.

Now it is relatively easy to obtain a sufficient amount of vitamin C in the diet. Good sources include oranges, orange juice, grapefruits, grapefruit juice, cantaloupe, strawberries, broccoli, brussels sprouts, and green and sweet red peppers. Fair sources include tangerines, tomatoes, honeydew melon, watermelon, asparagus, cauliflower, cabbage, spinach, and potatoes cooked in their skins.

For the cruising sailor with adequate food supplies—including citrus fruits, vegetables, tubers, and grasses—there is no need to take any vitamin supplementation. If food supplies are marginal, one multivitamin tablet per day provides a wide margin of safety.

The racing sailor must realize that because vitamins are used over and over again in metabolic reactions, the vitamin needs of an athlete are virtually the same as the requirements of more sedentary people. (The slightly higher requirement for B-complex vitamins is provided by any balanced, varied diet.) The racing sailor undoubtedly requires additional calories for energy, but not additional vitamins, minerals, or protein. For example, the average total daily energy requirement is about 2,100 calories for women and 2,700 for men. A 2,700-calorie diet formulated from the four food groups supplies the adult male with all of the protein, vitamins, and minerals he needs. If he engages in intense physical activity, he may expend up to 5,000 calories per day. The extra activity requires additional energy, e.g., 2,300 calories. Increasing the size of the portions, the frequency of the meals, or the variety of foods eaten at each meal can supply this additional amount. The importance of variety cannot be stressed too often. A diet composed of a variety of food sources obviates the need for supplementation of any kind, with the possible exception of iron (see the discussion of minerals next).

There is absolutely no scientific evidence that vitamins or minerals in addition to those available in a well-balanced diet improve health or exercise performance. In fact, the current "megavitamin" fad (doses up to 10 times the daily requirement) may result in serious harm.

Minerals

About 4 percent of the body is composed of a group of elements known as minerals. The minerals can be divided into the *major minerals,* such as calcium, phosphorus, iron, iodine, magnesium, sodium, potassium, and chloride (the last three known collectively as electrolytes), and the *trace minerals,* which, as the name implies, are present in minute amounts.

As with vitamins, mineral supplementation is generally unnecessary, because most minerals are readily available in a varied diet. The only exceptions are the electrolytes and iron. Electrolyte replacement and water balance are covered in depth in Chapter 3.

About 15 percent of women in the childbearing years have poor iron stores or iron depletion. Iron depletion does not mean that the person has or will develop anemia, although it may predispose to the condition. It does mean that the amount of iron stored in the body is less than normal. There is accumulating, but not conclusive, evidence that nonanemic, iron-depleted women may have a lower exercise tolerance than normal women. It is certainly true that iron-deficiency anemia *does* impair performance.

In most instances, iron stores can be augmented with a diet rich in iron, such as dried uncooked fruits, beans, peas, green leafy vegetables, egg yolk, liver, and kidneys. If it is documented (usually during a medical examination) that there is either iron depletion (and the woman is an athlete) or frank iron-deficiency anemia, then iron supplementation is required.

Calories, Exercise, and Survival

There is nothing mysterious about the relationship between calories and weight. Simply stated, body weight depends on only two parameters: the amount of calories taken in and the amount of calories expended in daily activities. Altering one or the other (or both) results in a change in body weight:

Stable weight	Calories in	=	Calories out
Increase in weight	Calories in	>	Calories out
Decrease in weight	Calories in	<	Calories out

That's it, pure and simple. It doesn't matter how the calories are provided nor when in the day they are taken in. All that matters is the total daily calories in and the total daily calories out!

The active adult man consumes and expends about 2,700 to 3,000 calories per day, the average active woman, 2,000 to 2,100. These figures are based on the assumption that a healthy, active person spends about 8 hours sleeping, 6 hours sitting, 6 hours standing, 2 hours walking, and about 2 hours in light recreational activities per day. Certainly, active sailors and sailing athletes expend more than that, but even athletes at the peak of training rarely consume and expend more than 4,500 to 5,000 calories per day.

A sailor who wishes to lose weight as part of a physical fitness program has three options. He can (1) decrease his caloric intake, (2) increase his activity, or (3) do both. It turns out that the third option is the most preferable since it results in the greatest loss of fat and the least loss of lean body mass, which includes the muscles and connective tissue.

Designing a weight-reduction program is simple. All you need to know is the conversion factor for calories and pounds of fat, which is approximately 3,500 to 1. Thus a net loss of 3,500 calories results in the loss of 1 pound of fat.

The most prudent rate of weight loss is about 1 pound per week. This requires a net deficit of 3,500 calories per week or 500 calories per day. One way to achieve this deficit is to limit intake by 500 calories per day. However, half an hour of moderate exercise (about 350 calories) performed three times a week produces a 1,050-calorie deficit; consequently, the weekly caloric intake need be reduced by only 2,400 calories instead of 3,500 in order to lose 1 pound a week. If the number of exercise days is increased to 5, causing a 1,750-calorie deficit, the food intake needs to be reduced by only 250 calories per day. If these 5-day-per-week workouts are prolonged to a full hour, then no reduction in food intake is required, because the 3,500-calorie deficit is created entirely through exercise.

If you want to arrive at an individualized approximation of caloric expenditure, see Table 5.2. This table lists by weight the number of calories that are expended per minute in a number of different activities. Simply

TABLE 5.2
Energy Expenditure in Various Athletic Activities*

				calories/minute for			
	110 lb	130 lb	150 lb	170 lb	190 lb	210 lb
Basketball	6.9	8.1	9.4	10.6	11.9	13.1
Bicycling 5.5 mph	3.2	3.8	4.4	4.9	5.5	6.1
9.4 mph	5.0	5.9	6.8	7.7	8.6	9.5
racing	8.5	10.0	11.5	13.0	14.5	16.1
Climbing hills (10 lb load)	6.5	7.6	8.8	9.9	11.1	12.3
Football	6.6	7.8	9.0	10.2	11.4	12.5
Gymnastics	3.3	3.9	4.5	5.1	5.7	6.3
Judo	9.8	11.5	13.3	15.0	16.8	18.5
Running 11.5 min/mile	6.8	8.0	9.2	10.5	11.7	12.9
9 min/mile	9.7	11.4	13.1	14.9	16.6	18.3
7 min/mile	12.2	13.9	15.6	17.4	19.1	20.8
5.5 min/mile	14.5	17.1	19.7	22.3	24.9	27.5
Squash	10.6	12.5	14.4	16.3	18.2	20.1
Swimming backstroke	8.5	10.0	11.5	13.0	14.5	16.1
breaststroke	8.1	9.6	11.0	12.5	13.9	15.4
crawl, fast	7.8	9.2	10.6	12.0	13.4	14.8
crawl, slow	6.4	7.6	8.7	9.9	11.0	12.2
Tennis	5.5	6.4	7.4	8.4	9.4	10.4

*Source: McArdle, Katch, and Katch, Exercise Physiology[10]

multiply the number by the duration of the activity in minutes. For example, a 170-pound adult who swam a fast crawl for 40 minutes would expend about 480 calories (12 x 40 = 480). There is one more step, however. If we did nothing but lie about all day, we would still burn up calories, through metabolic activity. The *basal metabolic rate* for men amounts to about 72 calories per hour (or about 1,730 calories per day) and for women about 56 calories per hour (or about 1,350 calories per day). Thus, the adult man who swam a fast crawl for 40 minutes would have burned up 48 calories if he had done nothing, so that his *net* energy expenditure is really 432 calories (480 − 48 = 432).[10]

The basal metabolic rate also becomes important during survival situations, explaining why food is so much less important to the shipwreck survivor than either clothing or water. A person rapidly adapts to starvation by reducing his basal metabolic rate from about 1,730 to about 1,200 calories per day, assuming that he does not engage in a great deal of physical activity. It turns out that the energy stores of the average man are about 81,000 calories—72,000 calories as fat, 8,000 as protein, and about 800 or so as carbohydrate. With these stores, a person should be able to survive approximately 67 days (81,000 calories ÷ 1,200 calories per day) before exhausting his energy supplies. In fact, this is about the survival time of adult men during famines or hunger strikes. Women, starting with more body fat, typically survive longer than men. By and large, recovery from starvation is doubtful after half the normal weight has been lost.

MARINE POISONS

Considering the number of fish that are caught and safely eaten each year, is there any reason for the cruising sailor to worry about eating his catch? From a strictly statistical point of view, there is probably not. But if you don't enjoy being a statistic, consider these two facts:

1. Marine poisons are, on the average, 100 to 1,000 times as potent as sodium cyanide.
2. Many of the world's most idyllic cruising grounds, such as the Caribbean and South Pacific, are replete with poisonous fish. On St. Thomas, poisonous species are so numerous that virtually all of the fish eaten in restaurants must be shipped in!

Although there are numerous types of marine poisonings, most of them are ones that the cruising sailor rarely encounters. The sailor need concern himself with three major types of fish poisoning (ciguatera, puffer poisoning, and scombroid poisoning), shellfish poisoning, and a few others.[11]

Fish Poisoning

Ciguatera

The most common of the marine poisonings is ciguatera. Although the syndrome was not described until 1787, it has presumably afflicted humans since antiquity. It almost prematurely ended the second Pacific expedition of the HMS *Resolution* under the command of Captain James Cook. The incident took place on July 23, 1774, at Malekula, New Hebrides. Cook and four crew members ate three fishes ("red pargo"), which are now believed to have been red snapper (*Lutjanus bohar*), one of the most common causes of ciguatera.

Ciguatoxic species are tropical or subtropical reef fish that either are bottom dwellers or feed upon bottom dwellers. Ciguatera usually does not result from fish that are caught in the open ocean; however, if these oceanic species do happen to wander close to shore and feed upon reef fish, they too may become toxic. Ciguatera is confined to a circumglobal belt that extends from 35 degrees north to 35 degrees south latitude. The most dangerous areas by far are the reef islands. Tropical reefs that fringe continental shelves (such as Florida) are also dangerous. Even within this belt, the geographic distribution is spotty. Fish from one sector of an island may be safe, whereas those from another a short distance away may be toxic. A region that has supported abundant safe fishing for as long as anyone can remember may suddenly suffer mass outbreaks of poisoning from a harvest of the same, previously safe species. Later, these species may revert to their nontoxic state, although this process often takes months. The cause of these rapid shifts is unknown. Sometimes they are associated with catastrophes, either natural (hurricanes, earthquakes) or manmade (wrecks, dumping, explosions), but usually there is no obvious triggering event. The relative unpredictability is particularly frustrating. In many places it virtually prohibits the establishment of shore fisheries.

The biogenesis of ciguatera is illustrated in Figure 5.1. There is unanimous agreement that the toxin—ciguatoxin—has its origin somewhere in the coral-reef food chain of herbivorous bottom-dwelling fish. The origin of the toxin has defied identification for many years.

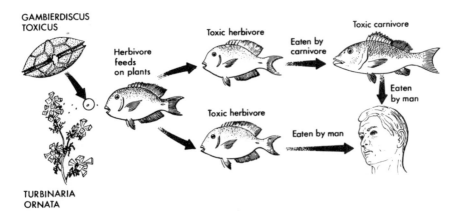

Figure 5.1. *The ciguatoxin food chain. Reprinted, by permission, from B. W. Halstead,* Dangerous Marine Animals (*Centreville, MD: Cornell Maritime, 1980*).

Previously it was felt that one or more strains of blue-green algae were responsible. However, the leading candidate at the present time is a new species of dinoflagellate (*Gambierdiscus toxicus*). The dinoflagellates are single-celled organisms that are a major constituent of oceanic plankton. They straddle the plant and animal kingdoms, possessing functions of both and prompting the name *plant-animals*. Herbivorous fish that eat the dinoflagellates acquire toxicity, but are themselves unaffected. Carnivorous fish become toxic by feeding on the toxic herbivores and are likewise unaffected. As a rule of thumb, the larger carnivores tend to be the most toxic because they can rapidly acquire large quantities of the toxin already concentrated in the herbivore. It is well known that the larger the fish, the greater the amount of toxin per unit weight and the greater the chance of becoming poisoned. The food-chain theory is supported by the fact that the most toxic portion of the fish is usually the liver, followed by the intestines, ovaries, testes, and muscle.

Over 400 species of fish have been incriminated at one time or another. The most frequently poisonous species are listed in Table 5.3.

The victim of ciguatera usually is aware of his intoxication within 3 to 6 hours, although signs may not appear for more than a day. There are two groups of symptoms: gastrointestinal and neurological. The initial symptoms are usually (60 percent) gastrointestinal, consisting of nausea, vomiting, abdominal pain, and diarrhea. Some victims, however, report muscle aching, cramping, and weakness as their first reaction. The next symptom is numbness and tingling in and around the mouth, in the throat,

---

TABLE 5.3
Species Responsible for Ciguatera

Most Common
Sea bass — especially grouper
Snapper
Jack
Barracuda
Moray eel

Less Common
Parrotfish
Surgeonfish
Triggerfish
Filefish
Porgie

---

and subsequently over the rest of the body. There may be "sensory reversal," when cold feels hot, and vice versa. Later on the victim may complain of headache or dizziness, or he may be confused. By the next day there is often intense itching and a rash. In severe cases, muscle weakness and incoordination become pronounced and are followed by convulsions, coma, and death due to paralysis of the muscles of respiration. Although the fatality rate had been as high as 12 percent in the past, most of the recent outbreaks have been more mild.

Except for some numbness, the symptoms in uncomplicated cases subside within 24 hours. Recovery from a severe ciguatera intoxication is typically slow, lasting weeks, months, and even years!

As of now there is no effective treatment. Induced vomiting is suggested to remove any remaining unabsorbed toxin from the stomach. Bedrest and painkillers are helpful. Hospitalization of severe cases is usually necessary but often not feasible because of remoteness.

Prevention therefore becomes crucial. Obviously, avoid all species listed in Table 5.3 unless you have good evidence that they are safe. In fact, the circumspect sailor should be wary of any species caught near shore in the ciguatera belt, since open-water species occasionally approach land and feast upon the indigenous reef species. Local knowledge is most helpful, but by no means foolproof. Natives actually make up a large percentage of all poisoning cases!

Despite numerous native folk practices, there is no reliable way to detect the presence of the toxin short of witnessing its effect on a living animal.

The appearance, smell, and taste of the fish are entirely normal. Ordinary cooking techniques such as frying, broiling, boiling, baking, and steaming have no effect on the toxin. Since the liver, intestines, testes, and ovaries have a higher concentration of toxin, these parts should be discarded.

A few native methods to test the toxin's presence are relatively reliable. Some tribes feed a portion of the fish in question to a pet cat or dog, and if the animal does not show signs of toxicity in a few hours (or better yet, overnight), the fish is eaten. A variation of this technique could be called trial by swallow or perhaps potluck. Since the degree of toxicity is related to the amount of fish consumed, one person can eat a small portion of the fish and wait several hours or overnight to see what happens. In the absence of any ciguatera symptoms, the fish is probably safe to eat.

The cruising sailor who wants to supplement his food stores can be quite fastidious in his selection. The castaway struggling for survival must live more dangerously. There are, however, some survival guidelines.

1. Unusually large reef fish, such as grouper, snapper, jack, or barracuda, should be avoided. Limit fish to under 5 pounds, preferably less than 2.

2. Eat only small portions of any unfamiliar fish.

3. Never eat moray eels. They are frequently *violently* toxic and can produce death in a matter of minutes.

4. Try to capture open-water fish.

5. As a last resort, eviscerate the fish and boil the muscle several times, discarding the broth each time. The toxin is somewhat water soluble. If that is not possible, soak the fish in seawater several times for periods of 30 minutes. This may leach out some of the poison.

Puffer-fish Poisoning

Puffer-fish poisoning is one of the most violent biotoxications. In contrast to ciguatera, however, it is a much more manageable threat to the sailor since all of the species implicated are members of a single order, Tetraodontiformes, which includes the puffers (globefish, blowfish, balloonfish, toadfish, and swellfish), the porcupine fish, and the ocean sunfish. These fish are all characterized by the remarkable ability to inflate themselves like a balloon by gulping down large quantities of water or air.

The geographic distribution of the Tetraodontiformes is extensive, from 47 degrees north to 47 degrees south latitude. Some of the species primarily inhabit tropical or subtropical reefs, whereas others, such as the sunfish, are open-water fish.

The problem of puffer poisoning is certainly not new. Egyptian tombs of the Fifth Dynasty (circa 2700 B.C.) depict the puffer fish *Tetraodon stellatus*. The accompanying hieroglyphics indicate that it was considered poisonous then as now. One of the Mosaic dietary laws (Deut. 14:9-10) was likewise directed at eliminating puffer fish from the diet of the Israelites: "These ye shall eat of all that are in the water; all that have fins and scales shall ye eat; and whatsoever hath not fins and scales ye may not eat; it is unclean unto you."

This would effectively eliminate all varieties of puffer fish as well as the oft-deadly moray eel, which causes ciguatera. It has been pointed out that essentially the same admonition was given to U.S. troops during World War II, 3 millennia later:

> All of the important fish with poisonous flesh belong to one large group, the Plectognathi [the former name for Tetraodontiformes], of which there are many kinds in the tropics. All these fish lack the ordinary scales such as occur on bass, grouper, sea trout. Instead these poisonous fish are covered with bristles or spiny scales, strong sharp thorns, or spines, or are encased in a bony boxlike covering. Some of them have naked skin, that is, no spines or scales. Never eat a fish that blows itself up like a balloon.[12]

As with ciguatera, the toxicity is unpredictable. The toxin, tetrodotoxin, has been well studied, although its origin in the food chain is still uncertain. The most toxic portions of the fish are the skin, liver, ovaries, and intestines. In contrast to ciguatera, where toxicity is related to size, small puffers are capable of packing a lethal wallop.

Tetrodotoxin is primarily a neurotoxin; gastrointestinal symptoms are usually absent. Within 10 to 45 minutes the sailor notices malaise, pallor, dizziness, and oral tingling that soon spreads to involve the entire body. Weakness and paralysis of the muscles of respiration follow. Death may occur in 15 to 20 minutes, and there is absolutely no treatment. If death occurs (and the fatality rate is 60 percent), it usually takes place within the first 24 hours.

If these fish have been identified readily since biblical times, why does puffer poisoning present any challenge at all? The sailor who eliminates all scaleless fish from his diet will never come into contact with the poisoning. Most cultures in fact consider all of the Tetraodontiformes to be "trash fish." But just to prove that "one man's fish is another man's poison," the Japanese (and to a lesser extent the Koreans and Chinese) consider puffer fish, which they call fugu, a delicacy! Because of the frequent outbreaks of poisoning—the fish is the cause of more deaths by poisoning in Japan than any other food—the government strictly regulates the sale and preparation of fugu. Fugu chefs are licensed, and there is even a cookbook on the safe preparation of the fish. However, as Halstead points out, it is "disconcerting to note that even the finest puffer cooks occasionally succumb to their own cooking."[13]

In survival situations, the fish should be immediately eviscerated and only the muscle eaten. Small pieces of the muscle should be soaked in water for 3 to 4 hours, during which the fish should be kneaded and the water frequently replaced. Since the toxin is water soluble, much of it can be leached out. Cooking has no effect on the toxin.

Since James Cook nearly lost his life to ciguatera (see discussion earlier in the chapter), one would assume that he would be more circumspect in his choice of fish dinners. Nevertheless, on September 7 (only 46 days after his bout with ciguatera), he very nearly succumbed to puffer poisoning! On this occasion, in New Caledonia, Cook and two of his scientific staff sat down to a meal containing a small amount of the liver and roe of a large puffer fish. All three men became severely ill and transiently paralyzed.

Scombroid Poisoning

Scombroid poisoning is the third type of fish poisoning of interest to the sailor. The name refers to the suborder Scombroidei, to which nearly all of the involved species belong, including tuna and such related species as bonito, mackerel, and albacore. Scombroid poisoning, unlike ciguatera or puffer poisoning, is a product of spoilage and subsequent bacterial contamination. The poisoning is not due to bacterial toxins per se. Rather, in the absence of adequate handling and refrigeration, several strains of marine bacteria interact with the fish flesh to produce *histamine* and *saurine* (closely related to histamine). These substances are responsible for the symptoms.

Usually—but not invariably—the toxic fish can be detected by its sharp, pungent taste. Symptoms develop within minutes and consist of intense headache, dizziness, abdominal pain, nausea, vomiting, dryness, burning of the throat, and difficulty in swallowing. Shortly thereafter comes flushing of the skin, itching, and hives. The face becomes swollen, the eyes red and watery, and the nose runny. In severe cases an allergic, asthmalike condition develops. Although deaths have occurred, the symptoms are usually transient, lasting less than a day.

Treatment consists of induced vomiting and the administration of antihistamines. In severe cases, epinephrine (Adrenalin) and steroids may be necessary.

Scombroid poisoning may be prevented by avoiding all tuna and related species not freshly caught or adequately refrigerated.

Paralytic Shellfish Poisoning

The biblical account in Exodus (7:19-21) of the Egyptian water turning into blood is probably the earliest record of what is now referred to as the red tide. This phenomenon results from the periodic proliferation, or "blooming," of dinoflagellates.[14] At least three species of dinoflagellates associated with paralytic shellfish poisoning have been identified: *Gonyaulax catenella, Gonyaulax tamarensis,* and *Gymnodinium breve.*

The process of paralytic shellfish poisoning begins when these toxic dinoflagellates proliferate and are ingested in large quantities by one or more of the filtering bivalve mollusks—clams, mussels, oysters, or scallops. The mollusk concentrates the toxin in its tissues but remains unaffected. Man completes the process when he eats the contaminated mollusk. The toxin in paralytic shellfish poisoning has been identified and labeled sax-itoxin, after the clam *Saxidomus giganteus,* from which it has been isolated.

Within 30 minutes of ingestion, there is a tingling or burning sensation of the mouth, lips, face, arms, and legs. In severe cases, tightness of the throat, difficulty in speaking and swallowing, dizziness, headache, pros-tration, muscle weakness, and incoordination follow. In the terminal phase the muscle paralysis becomes more severe, and the victim has difficulty in breathing (the usual cause of death). The prognosis is favorable if the individual survives the first 12 hours. Among 409 cases in a series of paralytic shellfish poisonings, the fatality rate was 8.5 percent, although recent cases reported to the U.S. Center for Disease Control were without fatalities. Two of these 55 cases did require respiratory support for a time.

Outbreaks of paralytic shellfish poisoning have occurred in various loca-tions around the world. The dinoflagellates tend to bloom in waters above 30 degrees north and below 30 degrees south latitude. Most outbreaks in the Northern Hemisphere occur between May and October, when the temperature of the water is the highest. Thus, the adage that cautions against eating shellfish during the months without an *r* has some truth to it, although September and October are also dangerous months.

The dinoflagellate *Go. tamarensis* is responsible for attacks on the eastern coast of North America (primarily Canada and Maine), whereas *Go. catenella* is associated with outbreaks along the Pacific coast (Alaska,

British Columbia, Washington, Oregon, and California). Other reported locations of outbreaks include the United Kingdom, France, Belgium, Germany, Norway, South Africa, Japan, and New Zealand. The red tide that occurs along both the Atlantic and the Gulf coasts of Florida is due to the dinoflagellate *Gy. breve.* Cases of shellfish poisoning off the Florida coasts have been mild, without paralysis or death.

There is no treatment except to induce vomiting. Thus, prevention is the key. Despite folk tales to the contrary, it is not possible to distinguish toxic from edible mollusks. As with fish poisoning, cooking does not inactivate the toxin.

It is important to differentiate paralytic shellfish poisoning from two other types of shellfish disease. *Bacterial shellfish poisoning* is a nonspecific food poisoning due to spoilage. The symptoms are due to the bacteria, not to the shellfish, so they are precisely the same as those of bacterial food poisoning acquired from other foods (see discussion in next section). *Erythematous shellfish poisoning* is an allergic reaction to the high iodine content of the shellfish. Within a few hours there is redness (erythema), swelling, and blotches over the face and neck, sometimes spreading to the rest of the body. The itching may be intense.

Additional Caveats

In addition to the common fish poisons listed above, some species of fish have toxic blood, others toxic roe, and still others have poisonous livers. As a general rule, *never eat the viscera (internal organs) of any fish.*

Bacterial food poisoning is caused by numerous bacteria and generally occurs either by infection or by toxins the bacteria produce. *Salmonella* is the most common example of an infection. Any food, especially meat, poultry, and dairy products, may transmit salmonella, or the foods may be contaminated by food handlers. After an incubation period of 8 to 48 hours, the victim experiences nausea, abdominal pain, and loose, watery diarrhea. Symptoms usually subside in 2 to 5 days. Antibiotics are usually not necessary. Although salmonella is relatively resistant to heat, thorough cooking kills most strains. Inadequate refrigeration of contaminated foods allows the organisms to multiply. Therefore, thorough cooking and prompt refrigeration diminish the chances. Avoid milk that has not been pasteurized! *Staphylococcal* (staph) food poisoning is due to contamination by food handlers. Pastries, custards, dairy products, and meats subjected to *improper refrigeration* are the common offenders. Symptoms typically appear 1 to 6 hours after ingestion due to a toxin the staph has already produced. The onset is abrupt, with severe nausea, vomiting, abdominal pain, and diarrhea. The symptoms last less than 24 hours, and no treatment is necessary. Cooking has no effect on the toxin once it is produced.

One other annoyance of which the cruising sailor should beware is the *parasitic diseases*. These diseases are especially prevalent in the developing areas of the world, which include many of our most idyllic cruising grounds! Freshwater fish are capable of transmitting both *liver flukes* and *fish tapeworm*. Beef is liable to harbor the *beef tapeworm,* and pork remains a hazard for both *pork tapeworm* and *trichinosis*. Fortunately, thorough cooking destroys all of these organisms. Smoking or marinating does not offer any guarantee of safety. Therefore, no matter how the sailor prefers his food at home, in foreign countries he should *eat all freshwater fish, beef, and pork well cooked.*

NOTES

1. S. E. Morison, *The European Discovery of America. The Southern Voyages* (New York: Oxford University Press, 1974), p. 174.

2. L. H. Roddis, *A Short History of Nautical Medicine* (New York: Hoeber, 1941), p. 127.

3. Ibid., p. 129.

4. Rum had been issued in the British navy since the early 18th century, initially at 1/2 pint per day. It was issued straight until 1740, when Admiral Edward Vernon ordered that it be diluted with water. The term *grog* has come to mean the mixture of spirits (usually rum) with water. Grog is said to allude to the fact that Vernon was known as Old Grog to his men, from the word *grogram,* a type of cloth from which his coat was made.

5. *Dietary Goals for the United States,* 2d ed. (December 1977). This document is available from the U.S. Government Printing Office.

6. Of course, there are always the drawbacks to be considered. In order to store glycogen, water must be stored as well, making glycogen a relatively heavy fuel compared to an equal quantity of calories stored as fat. Carbohydrate loading thus increases body weight slightly and may make the sailor feel uncomfortably "heavy." It is worth repeating that only racing sailors engaged in endurance tasks should use carbohydrate loading. The cruising sailor and the nonendurance racing sailor have no use for this technique.

7. Vitamins, minerals, and food supplementation now constitute a major industry in the United States. Rational discussion between the medical establishment and the proponents of various "nutritional therapies" is no longer possible. Either a person believes in them or he doesn't. By and large, the medical establishment (including the author) does not. The medical "party line" is that all of those bottles of vitamins, minerals, and food supplements are just so much movable ballast!

8. R. S. Allison, *Sea Diseases* (London: John Bale, 1943), p. 26.

9. Ibid., p. 28.

10. W. D. McArdle, F. I. Katch, V. L. Katch, *Exercise Physiology* (Philadelphia: Lea and Febiger, 1981), pp. 486-493. The reader is also referred to the forthcoming 2d edition of *Nutrition, Weight Control and Exercise,* by F. I. Katch and W. D. McArdle, published by Lea and Febiger, Philadelphia.

11. For additional information, see Dr. Bruce W. Halstead's excellent *Dangerous Marine Animals,* 2d ed. (Centreville, Maryland: Cornell Maritime Press, 1980), and *Poisonous and Venomous Marine Animals of the World* (Princeton: Darwin, 1978). The former is written for the layman and has a somewhat wider scope. The latter is more technical and encyclopedic.

12. Halstead, *Poisonous and Venomous Marine Animals of the World,* p. 2.

13. Ibid., p. 471.

14. Although red is the most common discoloration, plankton blooms may be yellow, green, brown, black, or milky-white.

6

Hazardous Marine Life

How strange, the tiger of the sea;
He runs from you and dines on me.

U.S. Navy, *Shark Sense,* 1959

THE WIDESPREAD INTEREST IN hazardous marine life is of relatively recent origin. It received its major impetus during World War II, when unprecedented numbers of men, casualties of downed aircraft or sunken ships, were forced to survive in the sea. This experience, coupled with subsequent biological research, has provided us with an abundance of useful information. The problem, however, is extensive. It turns out that most, if not all, of the major groups of marine animals include at least one species that is potentially dangerous to man. From a human perspective, the assortment of venomous spines, stinging cells, rapacious jaws, and other unpleasantries seems frightening if not downright malicious! But, of course, each of these characteristics represents nothing more or less than the owner's evolutionary adaptation to its particular niche in the underwater world. Human motives such as malice simply don't apply. The jellyfish, for example, could never have endured for millions of years were it not for its vast array of stinging cells. These stinging cells developed long before man was around to trespass upon the jellyfish's "turf."

The chances of contact with potentially dangerous aquatic animals increase as sailors cruise to remote areas of the world and begin to explore the beauty and wonder beneath the sea. It is clearly in our best interest to become aware of the physical characteristics that make some of these species dangerous. *We can then avoid inadvertently triggering an instinctive, reflexive response that was not meant for us at all.* Approaching the sea in a cavalier fashion is equivalent to walking alone down a dark alley in a strange part of town. It's asking for trouble.

ANIMALS THAT STING

The Coral Reef

One of the most popular marine attractions is the coral reef. Because the reef supports such an exuberant diversity of flora and fauna, it has been compared to a tropical rain forest; and like the rain forest, it harbors a great deal more than meets the eye. Although the lively and animated surface of the reef is readily apparent, there is a surprising amount of activity within the interior of the reef, out of view. In fact, many animals spend nearly their entire existence in the reef's honeycombed caves, crevices, and recesses.

Coral reefs occur in a circumglobal belt of warm water from 30 degrees north to 30 degrees south latitude. Despite its beauty, the coral reef itself represents a hazard to the unwary. The stony exterior belies the fact that it is an animal—or, more correctly, a colony of animals known as *coral polyps*. Each coral polyp sits within its own tiny cup of limestone that it erects by gleaning chemicals from the sea. The tiny, jellylike polyp retreats into its protective shell by day and hence is not visible. The brightly colored polyps can be seen only at night, when they emerge to feed, adding another chromatic dimension to the already multicolored reef.[1]

Coral cuts, lacerations, and abrasions are a major but generally avoidable nuisance. They usually result from careless swimming or snorkeling over shallow portions of the reef. Most people are simply unaware of the intrinsic sharpness of coral, as well as the increased vulnerability of wet human skin. Multiple factors determine the severity of coral cuts: (1) contact with the razor-sharp exoskeleton of the coral may cause a simple laceration; (2) microscopic pieces of the coral—calcium carbonate, sand, and other debris—retained within the abrasion or laceration may precipitate a "foreign body" reaction producing redness and inflammation; (3) bacteria, fostered by high temperature and high humidity, may infect the area; and (4) a weak venom that the polyp produces may cause swelling.

Since coral cuts may take months to heal (and frequently produce an unexpected scar), avoidance is the most prudent course. Never handle coral unnecessarily. Hands and feet should be well protected when swimming or diving on the reef. Divers should wear wet suits. If cuts, lacerations, or abrasions occur, they should be treated vigorously to prevent secondary infection and ulceration. Dr. Alexander Fisher suggests the following procedures:[2]

1. The lesions should be scrubbed with soap and water, using a soft brush or rough towel to remove any pieces of coral that may have become embedded in the wound.

2. Hydrogen peroxide should be applied and allowed to "boil" for several minutes. The wound should then be dried.

3. Isopropyl (rubbing) alcohol is next applied, and the contents of a tetracycline capsule sprinkled over the wound while it is still wet. This should be patted into a paste and allowed to dry. The crust serves as a bandage and will remain intact even after bathing. This allows the wound to heal from the outer edges. No additional bandage is needed.

4. If the wound does not heal promptly, it should be treated surgically, when feasible.

Jellyfish

Jellyfish are only very remotely related to the bony, or vertebrate, fish. They are invertebrates of the phylum Coelenterata, hence the expression "spineless as a jellyfish." Other members of the phylum include the true coral, false or fire coral, sea anemone, Portuguese man-of-war, and the hydroids. The basic structure of all of the coelenterates is a saclike body cavity (-coele) that serves as the digestive system (enteron).

In addition to the polypoid structure, coelenterates share another common feature, the *nematocyst,* or "stinging cell" (Figure 6.1). Each nematocyst consists of a minute capsule containing a coiled, hollow thread,

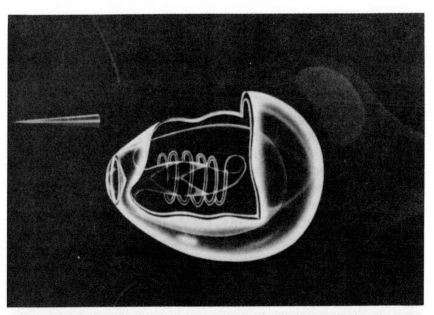

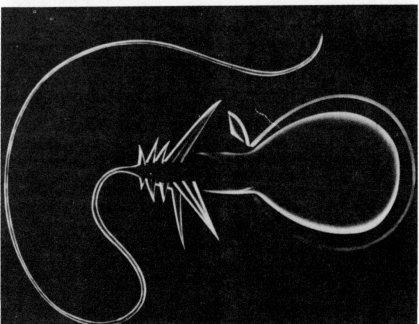

Figure 6.1. Nematocyst or stinging apparatus of coelenterates. (A) Undischarged nematocyst. (B) Discharged nematocyst. Note the coiled threadlike tube that conveys the venom. Semidiagrammatic. Reprinted, by permission, from B. W. Halstead, Dangerous Marine Animals (*Centreville, MD: Cornell Maritime, 1980*).

bathed in a venomous fluid. A hairlike trigger known as a cnidocil projects from the capsule. When activated, the cnidocil opens the capsule and the thread springs forth. Both mechanical factors (such as friction) and chemical factors (such as fresh water) seem to play a role in activating the nematocyst. Once the point of the thread penetrates its victim, the venom is released—a kind of tiny "hypodermic" injection.[3]

In most cases the jellyfish's reputation is worse than its sting. This is certainly true of most species of scalloped jellyfish, which periodically "bloom" during the warm, summer months. The common species include the "moon" jellyfish (*Aurelia aurita*), the "hair" jellyfish (*Cyanea capillata*), and the sea nettle (*Chrysaora quinquecirrha*). Contact with the tentacles of these species usually results in nothing more than a prickly or stinging sensation.

In stark contrast is the deadly sea wasp, perhaps the most dangerous animal in the sea! There are three closely related and similarly appearing genera: *Chironex, Chiropsalmus,* and *Carybdea*. Contact typically occurs when the victim is wading, swimming, or diving in shallow waters. The jellyfish may never be seen. Following contact, the sea wasp usually manages to tear itself away, but it leaves behind its calling card—a string of tentacles that resemble pink, purple, or grayish earthworms. The victim is usually in pain and attempts to struggle to shore. With extensive stings, he may lose consciousness and need to be dragged from the water.

The sea wasp's shape readily distinguishes it from the more benign species. In contrast to the scalloped hemisphere, the sea wasp is a cuboidal bell with flattened sides (Figure 6.2). Fortunately, its distribution is limited. The most dangerous species, *Chironex fleckeri,* is found almost exclusively in Australian waters, where most of the deaths have occurred. *Chiropsalmus quadrigatus* commonly inhabits the waters in and around the Philippines and has been responsible for a few deaths. The closely related *Chiropsalmus quadrumanus,* despite its wider range (including the tropical and subtropical Atlantic and Indo-Pacific), is much less toxic. Species of *Carybdea* are found worldwide, but have not been responsible for any serious reactions.

Jellyfish are feeble swimmers and are largely at the mercy of wind and wave. Incoming tides and storms are thus likely to bring the jellyfish closer to shore and increase the possibility of contact. Bathers should be forewarned that jellyfish washed up on shore are still capable of inflicting a serious sting. Even their detached tentacles have "live" nematocysts that can retain their stinging capabilities for up to 3 months.

The treatment of jellyfish sting depends upon the species. If the victim has been stung by the deadly sea wasp *Chironex fleckeri,* emergency first

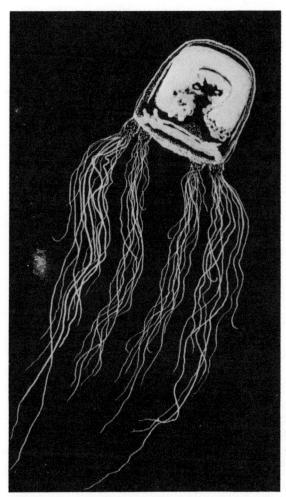

Figure 6.2. Sea wasp. Reprinted, by permission, from Thomas Helm, Dangerous Sea Creatures *(New York: Funk & Wagnalls, 1976).*

aid may be required. An antivenin with cardiopulmonary resuscitation should be summoned. An antivenin has been developed in Australia for the sea wasp and should be given if available.[4] At the same time, further absorption of the venom must be prevented. If an arm or leg is involved, a tourniquet may be applied. *No matter which part of the body is involved, the area should be flooded with any liquid that has a high alcoholic content,* such as drinking alcohol, rubbing alcohol, toilet water, cologne, or perfume. The alcohol inactivates the remaining nematocysts. It should be applied gently since friction causes the nematocysts to fire. Above all, avoid fresh water as it, too, activates the nematocysts. If alcohol is unavailable, meat tenderizer can be used as the primary treatment, although opinion varies as to its effectiveness. Once the above emergency procedures have been performed, the following steps should be taken:

1. After the alcohol has been applied, rinse the skin with a mildly alkaline solution such as baking soda in order to neutralize the acidic toxins.

2. If there are any tenacious tentacles, a paste of seawater and either baking soda or flour should be applied 5 minutes after the alcohol and alkaline treatments. The paste coalesces the tentacles, and they can be scraped off with a knife. In the absence of baking soda and flour, the tentacles should be wiped off with dry sand.

3. Tentacles should be removed only with a towel, stick, knife, or thick gloves—never with bare hands!

4. Don't allow the victim to shower in fresh water until all of the venom has been neutralized. Otherwise, the symptoms can be intensified and even cause shock.

If the victim is stung by a less hazardous jellyfish, he should follow the same steps except that the antivenin and tourniquet are not necessary.

Portuguese Man-of-war

Many people consider the Portuguese man-of-war a jellyfish, but it is a very different kind of animal. Unlike the jellyfish, the Portuguese man-of-war is a floating colony of different, specialized coelenterate polyps performing different jobs for the good of the aggregate. One type of polyp produces the bright blue (or sometimes red or green) float that bobs over the surface, while others lie beneath the float hanging head down, trailing long tentacles (Figure 6.3). The tentacles are armed with batteries of nematocysts similar to those of the jellyfish. The tangled mass of tentacles may reach 100 feet (30 meters) in length. Thus, a swimmer can be stung even at a great distance. The Portuguese man-of-war has no control whatsoever over its own destiny. It rests upon the water, its float acting as a sail, its tentacles as a sea anchor.

There are two species. A larger Atlantic species (*Physalia physalis*) is found in the tropical Atlantic, throughout the West Indies, as far north as the Hebrides, and as far east as the Mediterranean. The smaller Indo-Pacific species (*Physalia utriculus*) is found in Hawaii, Japan, and throughout the Indo-Pacific.

The Portuguese man-of-war has an undeservedly bad reputation! Con-

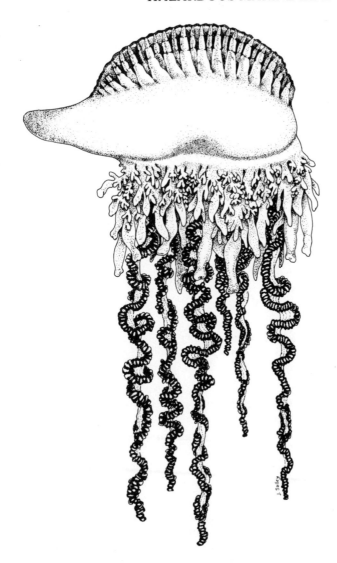

Figure 6.3. Portuguese man-of-war. Reprinted, by permission, from Bayard H. McConnaughey and Robert Zottoli, Introduction to Marine Biology, *4th ed. (St. Louis: The C.V. Mosby Company, 1983).*

tact with its tentacles produces the same pain and welts as the jellyfish and on occasion systemic symptoms also, such as muscular cramps and a feeling of chest tightness. However, death is extremely rare and is most

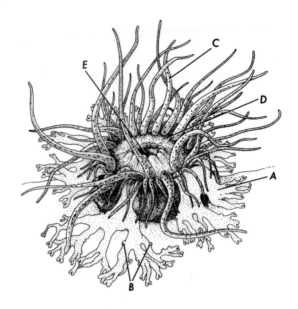

Figure 6.4. *Stinging sea anemone.* (A) *pseudotentacles with acrorhagi B;* (C) *tentacles;* (D) *oral disk;* (E) *mouth. Reprinted, by permission, from Frederick M. Bayer and Harding B. Owre,* The Free-Living Lower Invertebrates *(New York: Macmillan, 1968).*

likely to occur in either children or older individuals who sustain massive contact.

The treatment is the same as that for jellyfish stings.

Other Coelenterates

Since all coelenterates possess nematocysts, it is not surprising that quite a number of other species are capable of stinging man. Despite its appearance, *fire coral* (also known as false coral and stinging coral) is not a member of the true coral family. Rather, it is more closely related to the Portuguese man-of-war. Like true coral, however, it is widely distributed throughout the tropical seas of the Pacific, Indian Ocean, Red Sea, and Caribbean. The most dangerous of the fire coral is *Millepora alcicornis* followed by *Millepora dichotoma*. Both are so elegant that it is often tempting to break off a piece. A swift retribution follows in the form of a searing, white-hot pain.

Feather hydroid (Lytocarpus) is fairly abundant in tropical and sub-

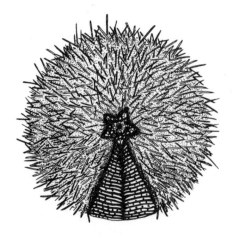

Figure 6.5. Sea urchin. Reprinted, by permission, from B. W. Halstead, Dangerous Marine Animals *(Centreville, MD: Cornell Maritime, 1980).*

tropical waters. Swimmers are most commonly affected while climbing onto offshore rafts or swimming around pilings. The feather hydroid venom produces one of two skin reactions: (1) weals that surface within minutes of contact or (2) a delayed chicken pox–like reaction 4 to 12 hours after contact.

Because of their variety of colors, animal *sea anemones* (Figure 6.4) are frequently mistaken for their botanical namesakes. Unfortunately, they are not as harmless. The severity of the sting varies greatly from species to species. Sometimes there is only a burning at the site of contact. With more severe stings, systemic symptoms may occur, such as headache, nausea, vomiting, fever, chills, and muscular spasms. Multiple abscesses, which are resistant to treatment, have also been reported. The sea anemone, like the fire coral, demands a "hands-off" policy!

Sea Urchins, Starfish, and Cucumbers

Nestling into nearly every nook and cranny in the reef is the ubiquitous *sea urchin*, aptly known as the living pincushion (Figure 6.5). Its body consists of a globular shell from which project calcareous spines. On the undersurface, in addition to the mouth, are short spines and tube feet, which allow slow locomotion across the ocean floor. There are numerous species of sea urchin, with great variability in the size and shape of the spines. Some species have blunt spines, whereas others have sharp, brittle spines up to a foot long resembling knitting needles. Most species are not venomous.

Sea urchin spines enter human skin with ease and can also penetrate leather or canvas gloves, shoes, and flippers. In some species a violet-colored liquid, possibly a venom, is released into the wound. The intense pain and burning create the impression of having stepped on a red-hot spike. The pain may last for hours if the penetration is deep.

Because of their extreme brittleness, once a spine penetrates the skin, there is a tendency for it to break off and become difficult to withdraw. If the spine cannot be removed, the body usually absorbs it in a few days. Occasionally, the spine must be removed surgically. Soaking in dilute acetic acid, boric acid, or even urine supposedly hastens absorption.

Closely related to the sea urchins are the *starfish*. Most of the starfish species are relatively safe to handle. One species, however, the crown of thorns (*Acanthaster planci*), possesses large spines and is capable of inflicting a painful wound. The spines are also venomous, which accounts for the occasional reports of numbness and partial paralysis. The crown of thorns can be found throughout the Indo-Pacific region. This species periodically proliferates widely: in the 1960s it laid waste vast portions of the Great Barrier Reef.

Cone Shells

Cone shells (Figure 6.6) rank among the most prized acquisitions of shell collectors. There are over 400 different multicolored species, one of which, the "glory-of-the-seas" (*Conus gloriamaris*), has commanded prices as high as several thousand dollars. However, the living cone shell is as dangerous as it is attractive. At least a dozen people are known to have died and scores have been injured by its venom.[5]

The cone shell surely possesses one of nature's most unique weapons (Figure 6.7). Tiny harpoonlike structures known as radular teeth are stored in a sac, like arrows in a quiver. These radular teeth are hollow and equipped with venom, which is stored in a separate venom bulb. When the cone shell prepares to strike, a radular tooth is transferred to the tip of the shell's muscular proboscis, which can extend several inches in all directions.

The victim experiences pain and numbness first in the area struck, but then over the entire body. Difficulty in speaking and swallowing and paralysis may follow. The cause of death is usually respiratory paralysis or cardiac failure.

Although species vary in toxicity, all live cone shells should be treated with caution and handled only with thick gloves. Supposedly, it is safe

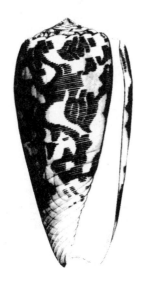

Figure 6.6. Cone shell. Reprinted, by permission, from B. W. Halstead, Dangerous Marine Animals *(Centreville, MD: Cornell Maritime, 1980).*

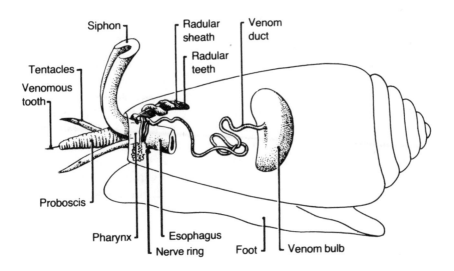

Figure 6.7. Venom apparatus of the cone shell. Reprinted, by permission, from B. W. Halstead, Dangerous Marine Animals *(Centreville, MD: Cornell Maritime, 1980).*

to pick up the cone shell by the "big end," but not always. The proboscis is quite extensible and may reach all the way back from the "little end" to strike the hand of the holder.

Immediate treatment consists of wound incision and suction. A tourniquet should also be used.

Octopus

Victor Hugo deserves much of the blame for the maligned reputation of the octopus. In his book *Toilers of the Sea,* he describes the octopus as "a disease embodied in monstrosity." Actually most species (including the large Pacific octopus, which has an arm spread of 30 feet (10 meters) and weighs more than 100 pounds (45 kilograms)) are not aggressive toward man.

Ironically, the most dangerous species of octopus is the smallest—the blue-ringed octopus (*Octopus lunulatus*). All octopuses have a sharp parrotlike beak, which they use to attack prey. Connected to the beak are two salivary glands that produce the venom. In most cases, the venom is not particularly toxic to humans. Usually a victim of octopus bite feels mild pain and a burning or stinging sensation. In some cases a spreading numbness and partial paralysis occur. The bite of the blue-ringed species, however, has caused fatalities.

Although there are a few closely related species inhabiting the waters around Australia, Japan, and the Indian Ocean, all of the fatalities, so far, have occurred in Australia. The species responsible is small enough to be held in the hand. Their speckled rings of blue often attract bathers, who have been known to pick them up and play with them! In fact, they are so small that the two tiny puncture wounds they inflict are sometimes overlooked. The venom must be extremely potent since, despite the small size, death from respiratory paralysis may occur within 2 hours. The immediate treatment is similar to that of cone shell envenomization: excision and removal of as much venom as possible.

Stingray

Stingrays cause more injuries to humans than any other venomous fish. Halstead estimates that there are about 1,500 victims per year in the United States alone. The many different species of ray are common inshore inhabitants of nearly all tropical, subtropical, and warm, temperate seas.

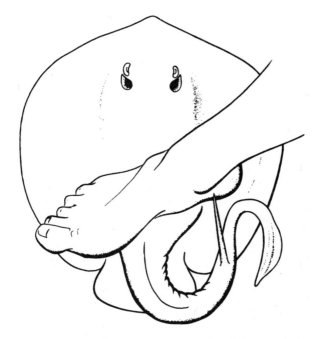

Figure 6.8. *Stingray inflicting its sting. Reprinted, by permission, from B. W. Halstead,* Dangerous Marine Animals (*Centreville, MD: Cornell Maritime, 1980*).

An additional reason for the large number of human injuries is the fact that stingrays are predominantly shallow-water animals. They frequently burrow into the sandy or muddy bottom, making themselves almost impossible to identify and a hazard to anyone who is wading through the water.

Although the stingray has a sinister appearance, there is no evidence of aggression toward man. In fact, quite the opposite is true. Virtually every attack is prompted by unintentional aggression on the part of man. In a typical scenario, the victim wades through the water and steps upon the stingray, often pinning it down. The creature's only defense is its venomous spine, or sting, located at the base of the tail. The tail whips forward, usually making contact with the victim's foot (Figure 6.8), although any portion of the human anatomy may be affected.

Pain is the first symptom, usually developing immediately or within 5 to 10 minutes. It increases in severity during the next 30 minutes and may spread to involve the entire leg. The pain is most severe by 2 hours and gradually subsides over the next 2 days. If the wound is deep and a substan-

tial amount of venom has been introduced, systemic symptoms may occur, such as vomiting, diarrhea, sweating, shock, paralysis, and, rarely,
death. The major problem is usually the wound itself and not the toxin.
There is apt to be significant tissue damage, since the sting has backward-
pointing teeth, which make its withdrawal a "nonsurgical" proposition.
The ensuing tissue damage increases the absorption of the venom, which
is contained along the side of the sting and covered by a sheath. When
the sheath is stripped away during penetration, the venom is exposed. A
sting that has been used repeatedly and not yet replaced may be so
traumatized that little of either sheath or venom is left. In that case only
the wound needs to be dealt with.

Treatment should be prompt. The wound should be irrigated with cold
seawater to constrict the blood vessels of the skin and reduce further absorption of venom. A tourniquet may be applied above the wound, but
it must be released for about a minute every 5 to 10 minutes to preserve
blood circulation. Next, the wound must be explored carefully for pieces
of the sting. Once the wound has been cleaned, it should be soaked in
hot water for an hour or so. After this, the wound may be closed and
antibiotics given if deemed necessary. Tetanus toxin, if available, should
be given.

Prevention is obviously the key. The chief danger, stepping on the
animal, can be largely eliminated by either shuffling one's feet along the
bottom or probing the area with a stick.

Sea Snakes

Sea snakes—all of which are venomous—are members of the family
Hydrophidae. With one exception, they are confined to the western Pacific
and Indian oceans. The exception is the yellow-bellied sea snake (*Pelamis
platurus*), which is widely distributed from the east coast of Africa to the
west coast of South America. This species reaches the western coast of
Central America and Mexico in considerable numbers (Figure 6.9). Sea
snakes have a distinct preference for sheltered coastal waters and especially
river mouths. Since they are air breathers, they are usually found in shallow
water.

Their disposition has long been a matter of dispute. There is now general
agreement that most species are usually docile, although if provoked they
may be aggressive toward man. Fishermen frequently are bitten while handling nets or sorting fish. Bathers may be bitten if they accidentally step
upon the snake.

Immediate treatment consists of suction of the wound (if it is within

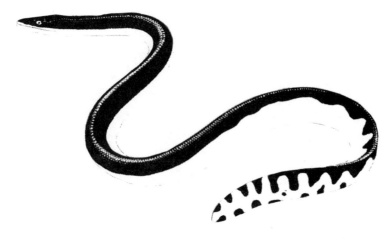

Figure 6.9. Yellow-bellied sea snake. Reprinted, by permission, from B. W. Halstead, Dangerous Marine Animals (*Centreville, MD: Cornell Maritime, 1980*).

a few minutes of the bite) and the use of a tourniquet (if within a half hour). The victim should be encouraged to rest and *avoid all exertion,* especially of the limb bitten. A sea snake antivenin has been developed and should be given according to the instructions. The antivenin can be obtained from the Commonwealth Serum Laboratories, Melbourne, Australia. It is recommended for anyone contemplating extended cruising in the Indo-Pacific.

Scorpionfish

Although a great variety of vertebrate fish have spines, only a small percentage possess a true envenomization apparatus. The most dangerous of these is the family of scorpionfish, which includes several hundred species. For convenience, they are divided into three main groups: the *stonefish* (*Synanceja*); the *zebrafish* (*Pterois*), also called the turkeyfish, or lionfish; and the true *scorpionfish* (*Scorpaena*). Despite some obvious differences in appearance, these species all have approximately 13 venomous dorsal spines in addition to an assortment of others. The venomous glands lie within grooves along both sides of the dorsal spines. In the stonefish, the glandular tissue forms two discrete, more highly developed glands, each with its own venom duct.

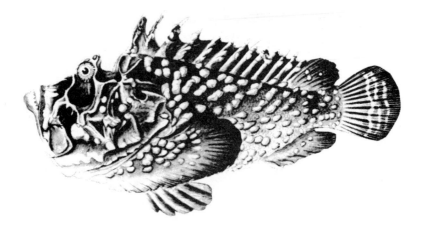

Figure 6.10. Deadly stonefish. Reprinted, by permission, from B. W. Halstead, Dangerous Marine Animals (*Centreville, MD: Cornell Maritime, 1980*).

The most notorious, and dangerous, of these fish is the *stonefish,* which has caused numerous deaths and countless injuries. The stonefish has a habit of lying completely motionless under rocks, in coral crevices, or beneath a layer of sand or mud. To abet its camouflage, it has developed the most incredible appearance (Figure 6.10). Its skin, which has a wartlike texture to begin with, becomes encrusted with bits of coral debris, mud, and even algae from continual burying in the sand. It looks for all the world like a piece of weathered coral or a chunk of stone, whence came the name. When it is stepped upon, the pressure forces the venom from the bulb along the duct into the wound, much like a hypodermic injection. The spines are sharp and strong enough to puncture even a thick rubber sole.

Pain spreads rapidly from the wound to involve the entire limb. In severe cases, the localized symptoms rapidly yield to nausea, vomiting, profuse sweating, delirium, convulsions, difficulty in breathing, and sometimes death.

Treatment consists of alleviating the pain, combating the effects of the venom, and preventing secondary infection. The wound should be excised and drained immediately. A tourniquet should be applied above the wound. Water as hot as the victim can stand should be applied as soon as possible and continuously for at least 30 minutes.

The development of a specific antivenin has made a profound difference in the outcome of stonefish stings.[6] For example, on the South Pacific island of Rarotonga, where stonefish stings are common, victims used to require hospitalization for several days. Since the introduction of the antivenin, hospitalization has usually been unnecessary.

Stonefish inhabit waters of the Indo-Pacific, Australia, China, India, and as far west as the Red Sea and the East African coast.

The *zebrafish* is as beautiful as the stonefish is ugly. This rather small fish, usually 3 to 10 inches (8 to 25 centimeters) long, is found adorning coral reefs throughout the tropics. It is often called *turkeyfish* because of its habit of spreading its fanlike pectorals and lacy dorsal fins, like a strutting turkey gobbler. This fish is truly fearless! If approached, it rotates its body to confront the intruder with erect dorsal spines. People are often tempted to grab this beautiful creature, especially when it lies motionless in the water. Invariably they receive more than they bargain for. There is immediate local pain. The tissues near the wound site become red and swollen as in a stonefish sting. In severe cases (usually the victim has received several stings), the pain is followed by nausea, vomiting, delirium, convulsions, respiratory paralysis, and sometimes death. The treatment is the same as for stonefish stings.

The *scorpionfish* comprise a more heterogeneous group widely distributed throughout all temperate and tropical waters, a few species even extending into polar regions. Unlike stonefish and zebrafish, some of the species of scorpionfish that inhabit temperate waters are of considerable commercial value as food fishes. For the most part, these species are bottom fish, preferring the rocky coastal regions—hence the term *rockfish*. The most common injury from these fish is to the hands of fishermen. The intensity of the sting varies from species to species, but generally there is at least an intense throbbing pain. The treatment is the same as for stonefish stings.

Weeverfish

The *weeverfish* are a group of small marine fishes confined to the east Atlantic and the Mediterranean. European fishermen have been aware of the venomous nature of these species since ancient times, long before most of the other venomous fishes were recognized. The weevers primarily inhabit flat, muddy or sandy bays. They bury themselves in the soft mud or sand with only their heads exposed, intermittently darting out to capture their prey.

Weevers each have approximately seven dorsal spines (plus a few other spines). Weever wounds produce instantaneous pain, usually described as burning, stabbing, or crushing. It is initially confined to the area of the wound but soon spreads to involve the entire limb. The pain usually subsides within 2 to 24 hours. The treatment of weever stings is similar to that of stingray wounds.

ANIMALS THAT BITE

Shark

Without a doubt, the most feared adversary in the sea is the shark. Is this fear justified? Well, yes and no! Certainly, unprovoked shark attacks do occur, causing mutilation and death. In fact, it is difficult to imagine a more horrible way to depart this vale of tears than by being eaten alive by a shark. But from a statistical point of view, the likelihood of such a death is quite small. There are only about 50 shark attacks per year globally, a figure that has remained relatively stable for the past few years. This estimate, however, is of *actual attacks,* whether provoked or un-provoked. *Encounters* are much more numerous, as any seasoned diver can attest. Most of the time a shark or sharks come over to investigate and, having satisfied their "curiosity," eventually depart.

Contrary to what you might expect, most victims live to tell the tale. Less than a third of shark attacks result in death. The likelihood of being killed by a shark is of the same order of magnitude as the chance of being struck and killed by lightning.

We are only now beginning to understand what makes a shark tick. That shouldn't be surprising, because when we are face to face with a shark we are really looking back across an abyss of time. The shark is a product of the late Mesozoic era and has changed but little in the intervening 300 million years.[7]

Of the 250 species of shark, only about 25 (or 10 percent) have been implicated in attacks on man. Except for the hammerhead, the name of which well characterizes its appearance, most sharks look very much alike to the untrained eye. The distinguishing features scarcely impress most swimmers and divers who encounter them in the water! Sharks range in size, at maturity, from 6 inches (15 centimeters) to over 50 feet (15 meters). Interestingly, the largest species, such as the 50-foot whale shark or the 45-foot (14-meter) Basking shark, are inoffensive plankton strainers, harmless to man. At the other extreme, many species are too small to cause any serious harm to man. Most of the species potentially dangerous to man are 7 to 20 feet (2 to 6 meters) in length, although it is a good general rule that *any* shark more than 3 feet (1 meter) in length *may* be dangerous, especially if there is food or blood in the water.

Most shark attacks occur between 45 degrees north and 45 degrees south latitude. The highest incidence is in tropical and warm, temperate waters above 68° F (20° C), partially because more people swim and dive in warm water. It is a myth, however, that sharks need warm water to attack. The most frequent period of the day for attacks is late afternoon and at night, which is sharks' most active feeding time; however, attacks may occur at any time. Generally, sharks attack people in one of the following situations: while swimming, while diving, or after surviving a sea or air disaster.

While Swimming

1. A swimmer is in the most vulnerable situation since he has neither warning nor defense. Obviously, stay out of water that sharks are known to frequent.

2. When possible, swim with a buddy or a group.

3. Never wade if you can swim, even in shallow water.

4. Avoid swimming in water when the underwater visibility is poor, or at dusk or at night.

5. Do not swim in the vicinity of garbage dumps. They are shark hangouts.

6. Before you enter and exit the water, first look around. Then move rapidly. The swimmer is most vulnerable at the surface.

7. Never enter or remain in the water with a bleeding wound. Women should avoid swimming in shark-infested areas while menstruating.

8. If a shark is encountered, begin to leave the area with slow, purposeful movements, rather than erratic, panicky splashing. Sharks are especially sensitive to low-frequency, irregular movements indicative of distress. If possible, face the shark at all times while making your exit.

While Diving

1. Never dive alone.

2. Always have assistance available. If you dive in known shark-infested areas, carry something to fend off an attack.

3. Wear dark clothing; bright, shining objects and contrasting shades tend to attract sharks.

4. If the group is threatened, form a tight circle and face the shark. Try to move steadily toward the boat or shore, but stay submerged until the last moment. If there are only two of you, stand back to back. If you find yourself alone, try to maneuver against a rock to protect your rear.

5. If attack is inevitable, the following maneuvers have occasionally

worked: releasing bubbles, shouting underwater, charging, clubbing the shark on the snout. For clubbing, use any object that is available, but use bare hands only as a last resort, since shark skin is quite rough and capable of inflicting severe abrasions—the last thing needed, since blood will attract other sharks and perhaps prompt a feeding frenzy.

For Survivors

1. Do not abandon any clothing, as it can afford some protection against the abrasive skin of the shark.
2. Remove wounded survivors from the water as soon as possible.
3. Remain quiet and conserve energy.
4. Do not dangle arms or legs over the side of the raft. You should assume that there are sharks in the immediate area—and there usually are. They are attracted to the raft by the fish that take up residence beneath it.
5. Do not fish when sharks are visible, and abandon a hooked fish if sharks congregate. Do not jettison garbage willy-nilly. Rather, save it on board in a container, if possible.
6. Despite the questionable value of Shark Chaser, a U.S. Navy repellent composed of a black dye and lead acetate, it should be used if available.

Finally, it is worth remembering that there are innumerable shark encounters for every shark attack. The odds are overwhelmingly in your favor.

Barracuda

There are about 20 different species of barracuda, which differ markedly in their aggressiveness toward man. This fact partially explains the conflicting accounts of the danger the fish presents. All barracuda are members of the family Sphyraenidae, and all are voracious carnivores; but the only species ever implicated in human attacks is the great barracuda (*Sphyraena barracuda*). Smaller species, which tend to travel in large schools, have never been known to attack man.

The larger specimens of *S. barracuda*, which look like large pikes, grow 6 to 8 feet (2 to 3 meters) long, weigh over 100 pounds (45 kilograms), and possess enormous knifelike, canine teeth. They are found in tropical and subtropical waters around the globe. Like all barracuda, they are swift creatures and hunt largely by sight. Unlike sharks, barracuda usually make only a single attack, which in most instances is not fatal to man. Mutila-

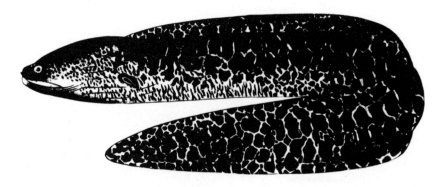

Figure 6.11. Moray eel. Reprinted, by permission, from B. W. Halstead, Dangerous Marine Animals *(Centreville, MD: Cornell Maritime, 1980).*

tion and amputation are not uncommon, however. Actually, there are only about three-dozen documented attacks on man by *S. barracuda*. Some have occurred when divers have towed dead fish behind them through the water, a practice to be avoided since it attracts both shark and barracuda. Some appear to be legitimate cases of mistaken identity, where the barracuda mistook the victim, or something he was wearing, for a more usual prey. Flashy metallic or multicolored clothes or gear may simulate the underbelly of a food fish. These attacks have usually occurred when turbid water impaired the fish's vision. In clear water, humans arouse little more than the barracuda's curiosity.

Moray Eel

Of the 20 or so species of moray eel (Figure 6.11), most inhabit tropical or subtropical regions, although a few range as far north as Europe. Larger species may attain a length of 10 feet (3 meters) and weigh as much as 100 pounds (45 kilograms). The moray is primarily a nocturnal creature. During the daytime it spends most of its time peering out from rock and coral crevices or pieces of wreckage waiting to grab prey that stray close by. Occasionally one is seen undulating across the ocean floor. At night it squirms out of its hiding place to hunt fish and octopus.

Whether by day or night, the moray eel almost never attacks humans unless provoked. Invariably an inadvertent poking of a hand or foot into the moray's lair or a direct assault upon the animal precedes an attack. Grasping or walking on the coral reef (not a good idea anyway) or feeling about inside submerged wreckage is an invitation to a vicious bite. In the

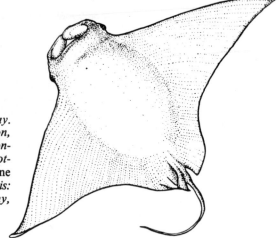

Figure 6.12. Manta ray. Reprinted, by permission, from Bayard H. McConnaughey and Robert Zottoli, Introduction to Marine Biology, *4th ed. (St. Louis: The C.V. Mosby Company, 1983).*

open water, however, when the moray does not feel threatened, it prefers to flee.

The moray is a notoriously powerful biter and can inflict severe lacerations with its narrow, muscular jaws, which are armed with strong, knifelike teeth. The wound is jagged and torn and readily becomes infected.

Manta (Giant Devil) Ray

The manta, or giant devil, ray (Figure 6.12) dwarfs the rest of the ray family. Specimens may attain a wingspan of more than 20 feet (6 meters) and weigh more than 3,500 pounds (1,575 kilograms). Mantas are generally found cruising or basking near the surface of the water. Inexplicably, they suddenly leap from the water and belly-flop onto the surface, producing quite a splash.

The manta is not at all aggressive toward man. Unlike its relatives, it does not possess a caudal stinging apparatus. It is dangerous only because of its huge size.

Needlefish

Needlefish are members of the family Belonidae. They have a svelte body that tapers into two elongated jaws filled with sharp teeth. Larger needlefish may attain 6 feet (2 meters) in length. Human fatalities and serious injuries are due to puncture wounds to the head, chest, and abdomen. These fish are frequently attracted to bright light at night and have been known to leap out of the water in its direction. Anyone standing in their flight path is liable to be punctured.

Needlefish primarily inhabit tropical waters. A person sailing or fishing at night with a bright light should be aware of this potential danger.

Giant Grouper

Giant grouper, or sea bass, as they are sometimes called, have occasionally caused problems for swimmers and divers. Some of the large species may be 12 feet (4 meters) in length and weigh over 500 pounds (225 kilograms). They tend to hang out in caverns, old wrecks, and underwater caves. Although they are not truly aggressive toward man, they sometimes pose a threat because of their huge size, curious attitude, and cavernous jaws. It has been suggested that Jonah must have been swallowed by a giant grouper, since whales cannot open their jaws wide enough to admit a man! The smaller specimens are as tame as puppies.

Killer Whales

The killer whale (*Orcinus orca*) has long been considered a ferocious and ruthless killer. It is about 30 feet (9 meters) when mature, swims fast, and has a formidable array of sharp teeth set within a powerful set of jaws. It usually travels in pods of 30 to 40 individuals and preys on a wide variety of marine life, such as fish, birds, walrus, seals, and even some of the other whales. It is quite capable of snapping a large sea mammal in half. But is it a maneater? Does it ever attack man? Roger A. Caras, in his book *Dangerous to Man,* has thoroughly examined the evidence and comes away unconvinced.[8] He marshals an impressive array of marine experts who support his contention that the killer whale is usually *not* a threat to man. If anything, the killer may be more of a threat to the boat than to man himself (small comfort, perhaps, miles from land). Two recent sinkings due to whales near the Galapagos Islands support this theory. Killer whales probably rammed and sank the Robertson family's boat, although everything happened so fast it is difficult to ascertain who saw what.[9] The boat sank in a very brief period of time, yet the whales made no attempt to attack the survivors. An injured sperm whale, not a killer whale, likewise attacked the Baileys' boat, making no attempt to molest them.[10] It is not known why whales occasionally attack boats. The act of feeding does *not* seem to prompt these attacks. Perhaps it is a case of mistaken identity (breeding rather than feeding!) or simply an example of cetacean psychopathology.

Giant Tridacna Clam

The giant tridacna, or so-called killer, clams abound in tropical waters. Claims have been made that divers accidentally stepping into the open valves have become trapped and have drowned. Actually, none of these reports is well documented. Since these clams close up tight with the slightest activity in the area, and close very slowly, many authorities doubt that it is possible that a man could ever become trapped. Dr. W. G. Van Dorn has stated, "Anyone so careless as to step into an open one while wading in the shallows along the Great Barrier Reef would probably deserve his untimely demise."[11]

NOTES

1. It is a great temptation to break off a piece of coral to take home as a souvenir. Don't! Not only will you irreparably mar the beauty of the reef, but you will also find that coral transports very poorly. After all, within the calcium-carbonate matrix there is living organic matter that will putrefy. The only coral that is proper souvenir material is dead coral washed up on shore. It can be recognized by the bone-white color, which signifies the absence of living polyps.

2. A. A. Fisher, *Atlas of Aquatic Dermatology* (New York: Grune and Stratton, 1978).

3. A number of factors determine the degree of hazard for man. In many species, the nematocyst is incapable of penetrating human skin, whereas in others it can penetrate with a vengeance. The toxicity also varies. True coral, as we have seen, does possess nematocysts, but they are not dangerous, producing at most a mild burning sensation. At the other extreme is the deadly sea wasp, *Chironex fleckeri,* which is capable of killing a man in less than 30 seconds. The amount of venom and the length of contact are also important. Although each nematocyst contains only a tiny amount of venom, contact with one or two tentacles of a jellyfish or a Portuguese man-of-war can easily activate thousands or hundreds of thousands of nematocysts—a formidable venom apparatus!

4. The Commonwealth Serum Laboratories, Melbourne, Australia, manufactures the antivenin for sea wasp stings. Anyone contemplating an extended cruise of Australian waters would be well advised to obtain the antivenin in advance.

5. A recent case is typical. A man was diving in Guam when he picked up a cone shell and put it in his shirt sleeve. He continued diving, never realizing that he had been stung. After an hour he felt numb and weak and was immediately taken to a hospital, but he died en route.

6. The Commonwealth Serum Laboratories also produces stonefish antivenin.

7. Sharks have been described as "beasts without a bone in their bodies or a brain in their heads," a statement not far from the truth. The skeleton of sharks (as well as of the closely related rays and skates) is composed entirely of cartilage without any true bones, a primitive but fuel-efficient arrangement. And although the shark brain is exceedingly small—and two-thirds of that is devoted entirely to the sense of smell—the shark more than compensates for any "intellectual deficiencies" with an exceptional ability to analyze and synthesize environmental stimuli.

For distances up to about 50 feet (15 meters), vision is the primary sensory organ. Ridiculous claims have been made in the past that the shark has poor vision, due in part to the myth that the shark has to be led to its prey by pilot fish. Pure nonsense. There is nothing to suggest that most, if not all, of the potentially dangerous species have anything less than excellent vision. Of course, individual sharks may be farsighted or nearsighted. Even so sublime a species as man is known to possess individuals with less than perfect eyesight. In addition to its vision, the shark's sense of smell is acute. It allows the detection of food or blood in the water at levels as dilute as a few parts per billion or less! Sharks are also endowed with taste buds and chemical skin receptors to analyze changes in the chemical composition of the water.

For distances greater than 50 feet, the shark depends on its acute sense of smell, its hearing apparatus, and a group of low-frequency-vibration detectors, which are sensitive to vibrations that a struggling fish or a person swimming might make in the water from as far away as a third of a mile or more.

There are two different types of feeding patterns common to most species. The first is the normal feeding pattern. Sometimes the movements are slow and determined, whereas at other times they are rapid and erratic. The final attack varies with the species and the circumstances. Frequently, a circling pattern around the victim presages the final attack, but this may be absent. When there is a sudden large quantity of food or a catastrophic event, such as an explosion, plane crash, or vessel sinking, a feeding frenzy—the second feeding pattern—may develop. Numerous sharks congregate and their movement becomes absolutely manic! They snap at everything in sight; cannibalism is frequent under these circumstances. The chances of a human surviving in the midst of a feeding frenzy are remote.

8. R. A. Caras, *Dangerous to Man* (New York: Holt, Rinehart, and Winston, 1975).

9. D. Robertson, *Survive the Savage Sea* (New York: Praeger, 1973).

10. M. Bailey and M. Bailey, *Staying Alive* (New York: McKay, 1974).

11. W. G. Van Dorn, *Oceanography and Seamanship* (New York: Dodd, Mead, 1974), p. 38.

7

Voyaging and the "Sea Diseases"

For the number of seamen in time of war who die of shipwreck, capture, famine, fire or sword, are but inconsiderable in respect of such as are destroyed by the ship diseases, and by the usual maladies of intemperate climates.

Scottish Naval Surgeon James Lind (1716-1794)

HISTORIANS OF SEAFARING have unflaggingly chronicled the heroic adventures and brave deeds of the nautical community. But for the common sailor, the perils of battle, storm, or shipwreck were minor compared to the danger of the "sea diseases." Until recent times, the sea diseases, or ship diseases, as they were also known, routinely decimated the sailing ranks. During the 18th century, for example, 1 in 7 sailors stationed in the Caribbean died annually of these diseases, and 1 in 15 was constantly on the sick list!

What were the sea diseases? The three major categories were *scurvy*, the *fevers*, and the *fluxes*. With the exception of scurvy, however, these disorders were not strictly associated with the sea. Even the early observers recognized that many were due to a "noxious land breeze." Today, most of these diseases would be classified as tropical diseases. Of course, until this century, the only way to get to the tropics was by sea!

Scurvy, a vitamin-C deficiency that afflicted sailors for hundreds of years, is discussed at length in Chapter 5. By the end of the 18th century, the Royal Navy had successfully mandated the routine use of lemon juice as an antiscorbutic.

The *fevers* included a number of communicable diseases that were not always readily differentiated from one another and so were grouped together. One of the most devastating of these fevers was typhus. It killed 2,000 men of the first English fleet sent to America in 1756. We now recognize that body lice transmit the disease. The 18th-century naval custom of sending out press-gangs to "recruit" the more unfortunate members of society guaranteed a constant supply of vermin-infested clothing, and the hideous overcrowding of ships assured the spread of the lice among the crew members.[1] Although typhus still exists (primarily in mountainous regions in the developing world), the risk for sailors is now minuscule. In fact, no American traveler has contracted typhus since 1950. The other fevers that posed a threat, and continue to threaten us, include malaria (previously known as the "ague"), yellow fever (or the "black vomit"), and typhoid fever (see discussion later in this chapter).

The *fluxes,* or diarrhea, usually afflicted men debilitated after long periods at sea or convalescing from one of the fevers or another illness. The outbreaks, which often reached epidemic proportions, were due to a variety of causes, including cholera, amebic and bacillary dysentery (shigellosis), viral enteritis, salmonella, and even staphylococcal food poisoning. Although the fluxes had a lower mortality rate than the fevers, they could be devastating. Soon after the defeat of the Spanish Armada, the English crews were so affected by acute enteritis that "many of the ships have hardly enough men to waie [weigh] their anchors."[2] Had this epidemic occurred somewhat earlier, this book might have been written in Spanish!

In recent times, the risk of acquiring illness generally depends on the area of the globe to be visited. Travelers in developing countries are at greater risk than those traveling in developed areas. In most developed countries, the risk is no greater than that incurred while traveling throughout the United States. Canada, Australia, New Zealand, Japan, and Europe are considered to be in that category. In Africa, Asia, South and Central America, the South Pacific, the Middle East, and the Far East, living conditions and standards of sanitation and hygiene vary considerably. Travel to major tourist areas entails less exposure to food and water of questionable quality and consequently a smaller risk. As sailors we frequently venture into smaller cities and towns off the usual tourist beat. Consequently, additional protection is often in order. This chapter contains specific recommendations regarding vaccination and prophylaxis for sailors traveling to various parts of the world today.

QUARANTINABLE DISEASES

From another point of view, all of the sea diseases (or tropical diseases) fall into two groups, depending on *whose interests are being protected.* The first group consists of quarantinable diseases, the second, nonquarantinable. Quarantinable diseases are those from which *various countries are trying to protect themselves.* From a practical point of view, the sailor is not likely to contract and carry any of the quarantinable diseases! The major reason for being vaccinated against them is to facilitate entry into a country. Without a valid vaccination certificate, you may be denied entry or be quarantined for 1 to 2 weeks, or more.

There are four diseases that the World Health Organization (WHO) considers quarantinable:

1. Smallpox
2. Plague
3. Cholera
4. Yellow fever

Smallpox no longer exists except in research laboratories. In 1980, WHO declared the world free of smallpox. This was 184 years after Edward Jenner performed his first vaccination in 1796 (the same year, by the way, that the Board of Admiralty ordered the use of lemon juice). The nautical community should take pride in the fact that the Royal Navy was one of the first to adopt routine vaccination, only 2 years later. Although WHO has recommended that countries no longer require an International Certificate of Vaccination against smallpox, Chad and Democratic Kampuchea still require one. A written statement from your physician stating that the smallpox vaccination is contraindicated for health reasons usually suffices and is recommended for these two countries.

The *plague* is now reported primarily in rural mountainous areas of a few countries in Africa, Asia, and South America. No country requires vaccination against plague as a condition for entry, so you don't have to worry about the plague either.

The risk of *cholera* to U.S. travelers is so low that it is doubtful whether vaccination is of any value. Unless the sailor goes out of his way to take food and water contaminated with infected fecal matter, it is difficult to obtain a large enough dose. Cholera vaccines currently available are of limited usefulness anyway. They have been shown to provide only about 50 percent effectiveness for a period of only 3 to 6 months. The sailor's best protection against cholera is to avoid contaminated food and water. The only reason to obtain a cholera vaccination is to satisfy the requirements of certain countries and avoid quarantine. Except for the rare outbreak, cholera is not endemic to the Western Hemisphere, so if your travels are restricted to this hemisphere, do not even bother with the cholera vaccination. The same applies to the rest of the developed countries. However, if your itinerary includes or might include any countries in Africa or Asia, it is easiest to go ahead and obtain the vaccination. A single dose of vaccine will satisfy international health regulations.

The same kind of logic applies to the *yellow fever* vaccination. There are yellow fever endemic zones in Africa and South America. From these zones outbreaks of yellow fever have occurred in the last few decades— although, at any one time, most countries are free of yellow fever! In fact, international health regulations no longer recognize endemic zones. Nevertheless, many countries in the world continue to use this concept and will consider you potentially infectious if you have visited an endemic area, *whether or not it is currently infected.* Thus, if you plan to visit any of these countries, it is probably wise to obtain the vaccination. It provides protection for more than 3 years.

NONQUARANTINABLE DISEASES

The nonquarantinable diseases are those that various countries already have. *It is entirely up to the individual to avoid contracting them.*

Malaria is a nonquarantinable disease caused by several species of *Plasmodium,* a parasite that infects red blood cells. It is usually transmitted from human to human through the bite of an infected anopheles mosquito. Headache, malaise, fever, chills, and sweats, which may occur at intervals, are symptoms of the disease. There may be anemia and jaundice, and in the case of one malarial species, *Plasmodium falciparum,* even heart or kidney failure, coma, and death. Deaths due to malaria are preventable. Everyone, regardless of age, who enters an area where the risk exists for malaria transmission should take prophylactic medication, *even for visits as brief as one night.*

Areas where malaria is known to exist include parts of Mexico, Haiti, Central America, South America, Africa, the Middle East, Turkey, the

Indian subcontinent, Southeast Asia, the People's Republic of China, the Indonesian archipelago, and Oceania. There is no malaria risk in North America, Europe, Australia, New Zealand, and Japan. The risk of acquiring disease is not uniform from country to country or even within countries, and it frequently changes from year to year. It depends on local conditions such as mosquito density, prevalence of infection, weather, and altitude. Since the pattern of malaria changes frequently, available information should be used with caution. Occasionally, contradictory information is reported from different sources. When in doubt, it is better to err on the side of caution by taking prophylactic medication.

In most areas, chloroquine phosphate (Aralen) is the drug of choice (see Table 7.1). To date only certain strains of *P. falciparum* in specific geographic areas are resistant to chloroquine. Travelers to a few regions of South America, Panama, the Indian subcontinent, Southeast Asia, the Indonesian archipelago, the Philippines, New Guinea, and East Africa are at risk (Table 7.2). An effective drug for the suppression of chloroquine-resistant *P. falciparum,* in areas where such strains are widespread, is a fixed combination of pyrimethamine and sulfadoxine (Fansidar, Falcidar) (Table 7.1). This combination should always be taken *in addition to* chloroquine, the preferred drug for the suppression of the other malarious strains, such as *P. vivax* and *P. ovale.*

In addition to taking antimalaria medication, exposure to mosquitoes should be avoided by sleeping inside well-screened areas or under mosquito netting. Outdoors, exposure can be reduced by wearing clothing that adequately covers the arms and legs, by periodic application of mosquito repellents, and by reducing outdoor activities in the evening when malarious mosquitoes usually bite. The most effective repellent is N, N-Diethyl-meta-toluamide (deet), an ingredient in many commercially available insect repellents.[3]

Typhoid vaccination is not required for international travel, but it is recommended for travelers to areas where there is a recognized risk of exposure because of poor food and water sanitation. Typhoid is prevalent in many countries of Africa, Asia, and Central and South America. The typhoid vaccine has been shown to protect 70 to 90 percent of recipients, depending in part on the degree of subsequent exposure. However, even those who have been vaccinated should use caution in selecting food and water (see discussion later in this chapter).

Tetanus remains an important health problem. Since there is no natural immunity to the tetanus toxin and since the tetanus organism is found throughout the world, it is imperative to have primary immunization with a booster every 10 years. Most cases of *diphtheria* occur in unimmunized

TABLE 7.1
Dosages of Antimalaria Drugs

Generic name	Brand name	Adult dose	Pediatric dose	Formulations[3]
Chloroquine phosphate[1]	*Aralen* *Avlochlor* *Resochin* many others	300 mg base (500 mg salt) once weekly 1–2 weeks prior to, during, and 6 weeks after exposure	5 mg base (8.3 mg salt) per kg once weekly not to exceed adult dose	Tablets: 150 mg base (250 salt) 300 mg base (500 salt) other preparations [base 37.5, 50, 75, 100 mg] Syrup: [25 and 50 mg base/5 ml]
Hydroxychloroquine[2]	*Plaquenil* *Ercoquin* *Quensyl*	310 mg base (400 mg salt) once weekly 1–2 weeks prior to, during, and 6 weeks after exposure	5 mg base (6.5 mg salt) per kg once weekly not to exceed adult dose	Tablets: 155 mg base (200 salt)
Chloroquine sulfate[2]	*Nivaquine* *Bemasulph*	300 mg base (410 mg salt) once weekly during and for 6 weeks after exposure	5 mg base (6.8 mg salt) per kg once weekly not to exceed adult dose	Tablets: [100 mg base (137 salt)] [146 mg base (200 salt)] Syrup: [25 mg base (34 salt)/ml] [50 mg base (68 salt)/ml]
Amodiaquine[2]	*Camoquin* *Flavoquine* *Basoquin*	400 mg base (520 mg salt) once weekly during and for 6 weeks after exposure	7 mg base (9 mg salt) per kg once weekly not to exceed adult dose	Tablets: [200 mg base (260 salt)] Powder: [150 mg base/5 ml]
Pyrimethamine-sulfadoxine	*Fansidar* *Falcidar*	25 mg pyrimethamine and 500 mg sulfadoxine (1 tablet) once weekly during and for 6 weeks after exposure	Weekly: 4–10 kg = 1/8 tablet 10–15 kg = 1/4 tablet 15–30 kg = 1/2 tablet 30–50 kg = 3/4 tablet 50 kg = 1 tablet	Combination tablet: 25 mg pyrimethamine and 500 mg sulfadoxine

[1]drug of choice
[2]alternative drugs
[3]formulations in brackets not available in U.S.

TABLE 7.2
Areas with Chloroquine-Resistant Malaria

Bangladesh
Brazil (interior and coastal area north of Rio de Janeiro)
China, People's Republic of (parts)
Colombia (all malarious areas; in general, all except Bogota and environs)
Democratic Kampuchea
Ecuador (interior bordering Colombia)
French Guiana (isolated reports)
Guyana (interior)
India (mostly areas north and east of Bangladesh)
Indonesia (E. Kalimantan — Island of Borneo, Irian Jaya)
Kenya (recent cases)
Lao People's Republic
Madagascar (recent cases)
Malaysia
Panama (all malarious areas east of Canal Zone including San Blas Islands)
Papua New Guinea
Philippines (many regions)
Solomon Islands
Surinam
Tanzania (recent cases)
Uganda (recent cases)
Venezuela
Vietnam

or inadequately immunized individuals. Adequate immunization offers protection for 10 years or more. Many sailors have received the DTP vaccine (diphtheria-tetanus-pertussis) in childhood. A booster injection of adult type Td (tetanus-diphtheria) is all that is needed. If the sailor has never been immunized, a three-dose series is recommended.

Poliomyelitis is no longer a significant hazard in westernized countries due to the effective use of vaccines during the past 3 decades. However, recent evidence suggests that its incidence is actually on the *increase* in many parts of the developing world. Because the length of protection that the primary series provides is unknown, it is prudent to obtain a booster vaccination prior to embarkation. This protects the sailor for at least 5 years, probably much more. If the oral polio vaccine (OPV, Sabin) was used for the primary course, one additional dose of OPV should be used. If inactivated polio vaccine (IPV, Salk) was used for the primary series, either OPV or IPV can be used.[4] If the sailor has never been immunized, he should *definitely* receive the primary series prior to shipping out.

There are two major forms of *hepatitis,* A and B. Hepatitis A (formerly known as infectious hepatitis) constitutes a risk for travelers to areas of the world where it is endemic, especially Africa and Asia. Sailors are generally at higher risk since they routinely bypass the usual tourist routes. Brief stopovers probably require no protection, but anyone planning to stay 3 or more months in tropical areas or developing countries would benefit from the prophylactic use of immune globulin. It offers at least partial protection against hepatitis A (and probably some against hepatitis B as well) for 4 to 6 months. Because the protection is short-lived, repeated doses may be necessary. Fortunately, immune globulin can be obtained in most countries. Uncooked items, especially raw shellfish such as clams and oysters, have been responsible for some outbreaks, so they should be avoided. A vaccine for hepatitis B has recently been approved in the United States, but routine use for travelers has not been recommended.

TRAVELER'S DIARRHEA

Taking on water in a foreign port worries most sailors. One reason is the common, but largely avoidable, problem of traveler's diarrhea (the "flux"), which is prevalent around the world, particularly in developing, nonwesternized countries.

A number of different organisms, including bacteria, viruses, and even parasites (amebiasis, giardiasis), cause diarrhea. Most commonly it is due to strains of bacteria with which the sailor's gastrointestinal (GI) tract is not familiar. These strains are indigenous to a particular area, and the local inhabitants have adapted to them. In Mexico, for example, certain strains of the common bacteria *E. coli* (different from those that normally colonize our GI tract) most often cause traveler's diarrhea. In other ports of call, different foreign strains are responsible. What is common to all of these bacteria is that they elaborate a toxin similar in its effect to the toxin that cholera produces (although not as powerful). This toxin causes a loss of water and electrolytes (sodium, chloride, potassium, and bicarbonate) from the GI tract, resulting in diarrhea.

There are a number of simple, practical methods of purifying and disinfecting water to prevent traveler's diarrhea. Vigorous boiling for 5 minutes is the most reliable method but is only practical for small quantities of water. After boiling, allow the water to cool to room temperature—do not add ice! (Adding a pinch of salt per quart, or pouring the water several times from one container to another, improves the taste.) Commercial tablets, such as Halazone, are available but are expensive.

TABLE 7.3
Treatment of Water with Chlorine

	Drops* to be added per quart or liter	
Available chlorine	Clear water	Cold or cloudy water**
1%	10	20
4%–6%	2	4
7%–10%	1	2
Unknown	10	20

*1 drop = 0.05 ml. Mix thoroughly by stirring or shaking water in container. Let stand for 30 minutes. A slight chlorine odor should be detectable in the water; if not, repeat the dosage and let stand for another 15 minutes before using. Water is safe to use.

**Very turbid or cold water may require prolonged contact time; let stand up to several hours prior to use, if possible.

The least expensive method is to add liquid chlorine such as that found in laundry bleach (Table 7.3). After mixing, allow the water to stand for 30 minutes. If there is not a slight chlorine odor, repeat the process and wait another 15 minutes. The water is then safe to use. The chlorine taste dissipates once the vessel is underway (due to the increased aeration of the water). Swimming pool chlorine is also effective at a dose of about ½ teaspoon per 100 gallons. Once again, repeat the dose if there is not a slight chlorine odor. If chlorine is not available, tincture of iodine is also effective (Table 7.4). After a 30-minute wait, the water is safe to drink.

Remember that if water is contaminated, ice made from that water must also be considered unsafe. Alcohol, incidentally, does not "purify" contaminated water or ice. Neither does bottling per se, unless the bottled liquid is also sterilized (which is often impossible to ascertain). On the whole, uncarbonated bottled beverages (water, fruit drinks, and so forth) should be considered suspect. However, carbonated bottled water, other carbonated beverages, and alcoholic beverages when taken straight are usually safe to drink. So is tea or coffee made with boiled water.

It is safer to drink directly from a beverage can or bottle than from a questionable container. But water on the outside of cans or bottles might be contaminated. Therefore, wet cans or bottles should be dried before opening and the surfaces that are in direct contact with the mouth should be wiped clean.

Raw fruits that you peel yourself are generally safe to eat; raw, leafy

TABLE 7.4
Treatment of Water with Tincture of Iodine

| Tincture of iodine (from medicine chest or first-aid kit) | Drops* to be added per quart or liter | |
	Clear water	Cold or cloudy water**
2%	5	10

*1 drop = 0.05 ml. Let stand for 30 minutes. Water is safe to use.

**Very turbid or cold water may require prolonged contact time; let stand up to several hours prior to use, if possible.

vegetables should be avoided, however, until first disinfected in a chlorine solution. In a pinch, soaking in vinegar water (of high concentration) will kill everything except parasitic cysts.

Although these practices do not absolutely guarantee immunity from traveler's diarrhea, they markedly reduce the risk. They are also of proven value in the prevention of more serious infections, such as cholera, typhoid, and shigellosis.

The sailor who, despite his best efforts, contracts traveler's diarrhea should be aware of some of the newer concepts in treatment. First, unless there is blood or pus in the stool, antibiotics are probably not necessary. Second, opinion is currently in a state of flux regarding the value of antimotility, or antispasmodic, drugs, such as paregoric or diphenoxylate hydrochloride (Lomotil). It used to be felt that if the purging process could be controlled, the patient would quickly recover. A more recent approach holds that diarrhea is nature's way of ridding the body of both the toxin(s) and the bacteria that produce it (them); as a result, diarrhea should be allowed to continue, *provided the fluid can be replaced.* If antidiarrhea agents are used, they should be used with caution and never for more than 2 to 3 days. Persons with fever or blood or mucus in the stools should not use them. Kaolin-pectin preparations (e.g., Kaopectate, U.S.) may alter stool consistency, but they do not modify the illness. Bismuth subsalicylate (Pepto-Bismol, U.S.) may be of value in preventing and treating diarrhea in adults. In a study of its use for prevention in adults, high-dose Pepto-Bismol was successful in decreasing the diarrhea. Unfortunately, the dosage is high, so it is impractical to carry enough Pepto-Bismol for either prevention or treatment.

Third, and most important, studies have shown that oral rehydration

---

TABLE 7.5
Oral Rehydration for Acute Diarrhea

Prepare two separate glasses with the following ingredients:

Number 1

Fruit juice (e.g., orange, apple) This is rich in potassium.	8 ounces

Honey or corn syrup
  This contains the glucose essential
  for absorption.
	1/2 teaspoon

Table salt Table salt is sodium chloride.	1 pinch

Number 2

Water (carbonated or boiled)	8 ounces
Baking soda This contains sodium bicarbonate.	1/4 teaspoon

Drink alternately from each glass. Water, tea, or carbonated beverages can supplement, but most of the replacement fluids should be from glasses Number 1 and Number 2.

---

is an effective method to replace all of the lost water and electrolytes. Formerly, it was possible to replace fluids only intravenously, since fluid taken orally was not absorbed and only added to the diarrhea. It is now known, however, that the GI tract can absorb all of the necessary water and electrolytes, *provided the oral solution contains glucose!* Commercial prepackaged, powdered preparations of such a solution developed by the World Health Organization are available in most countries. This formula contains potassium chloride, 1.5 grams per liter; sodium chloride, 3.5 grams per liter; sodium bicarbonate, 2.5 grams per liter; and glucose, 20 grams per liter. Table 7.5 gives a simple, recommended home formula for the treatment of diarrhea, which can be prepared from ingredients available on most vessels. Table 7.6 lists four additional formulas that do just about the same thing.

Finally, the routine prophylactic use of antibiotics is not recommended because of possible side effects and the likelihood of inducing resistance. Antibiotics reduce the protective effect of a person's own bacterial flora. Doxycycline (Vibramycin), a tetracyclinelike drug, has been recommended in some quarters and may be of value when dealing with *E. coli*

TABLE 7.6
Alternative Methods for Rehydration

I.   4 tbsp sugar (45 gm),
     or 3 tbsp honey/Karo
     3/4 tsp salt (4 gm NaCl)
     1 tsp baking soda (4 gm NaHCO₃)
     1 c orange juice
     add water to make 1 liter

II. 1 3-oz pkg Jell-O
     1 tsp baking soda

III. 1 bouillon cube
     2/3 tsp baking soda
     4 tbsp sugar
     add water to make 1 liter

IV. Gatorade or any other electrolyte drink is fine. All you need
     to do is add 4 tbsp sugar per liter.

---

organisms, which are susceptible to it. However, in some areas *E. coli* are not sensitive to doxycycline. Side effects of the drug, such as extreme sensitivity to sunlight, may occur, and the use of the drug may increase the likelihood of a person acquiring more serious GI infections that organisms unresponsive to doxycycline may cause.

MISCELLANEOUS HEALTH HINTS

1. Avoid swimming in freshwater lakes, streams, and ponds. Three closely related species of blood flukes produce a disease known as *schistosomiasis*. Another, albeit less likely, possibililty is *amebic meningoencephalitis*.

2. Wear shoes when walking in sandy soil—beware of the *hookworm*.

3. Travelers to the Caribbean are advised not to purchase Haitian goatskin handicrafts. They have been found to contain *anthrax* spores. Anthrax is caused by a bacterial organism that produces spores highly resistant to disinfection. These spores may persist in a contaminated item for many years.

NOTES

1. There was a perverse logic in the once-common practice of overcrowding. Because the sea diseases *routinely* decimated the crew, extra bodies theoretically

did not have to be carried aboard to take their place. It was not realized until much later that overcrowding actually *hastened* the spread of these diseases.

2. L. H. Roddis, *A Short History of Nautical Medicine* (New York: Hoeber, 1941), p. 125.

3. Cutter's is one of the most popular and effective brands of insect repellent.

4. IPV is somewhat difficult to obtain. It is recommended for unvaccinated adults, since there is a minor risk of acquiring polio from OPV.

8

Sailing Vision

The sea never changes, and its
works, for all the talk of men,
are wrapped in mystery.

Joseph Conrad, *Typhoon*, 1902

IMAGINE YOURSELF IN A pea-soup fog on a moonless night off a lee shore. What is your response? Well, depending on your experience, it falls somewhere between anxiety and terror! We can never feel entirely at ease on the water when deprived of our most valuable sense—vision. It doesn't matter how much we surround ourselves with modern electronic gadgetry; we are never comfortable until we can *see* the lighted buoy that marks the shoal or channel. This example serves to highlight the preeminence of vision in the day-to-day life of every mariner, be he racer or cruiser, weekender or circumnavigator. From spotting a cat's-paw or a buoy to finding the entrance to a coral reef, sailing is foremost a visual activity.

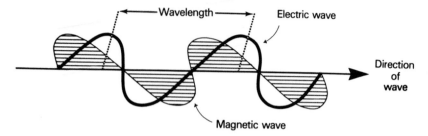

Figure 8.1. Electromagnetic wave.

Despite the preeminence of vision, few sailors are familiar with anything but the rudiments of the visual system. This is doubly unfortunate. First, the system is both sensitive and sophisticated, and the better we understand it, the more of its untapped resources we can use. Second, since it is sophisticated, we must be on guard lest we misunderstand what it is telling us. These misunderstandings or visual illusions are particularly common on the water.

THE GRAND SPECTRUM

Although we don't usually think about it, light has a precise definition. Light is energy from a specific portion of the *electromagnetic spectrum* that is capable of stimulating the retina of the human eye.[1] To be precise, the human eye is only sensitive to radiation with wavelengths between about 400 and 700 nanometers. (A nanometer is one-billionth of a meter.) Radiation of longer wavelengths comprises the infrared band, whereas shorter wavelengths produce ultraviolet radiation (see Figure 4.1). There is no a priori reason why the human eye should be limited to this narrow band. Infrared, ultraviolet, and even X-ray vision are within nature's technical capabilities. There is, however, a simple evolutionary explanation. The wavelengths we perceive as light are maximally transmissible through water; shorter and longer wavelengths simply do not travel through water very well. Since our oceanic ancestors were not exposed to much infrared or ultraviolet radiation, there was no reason to develop receptors sensitive to either. Although the spectrum has shifted slightly since we came ashore and "dried out," by and large we respond to the same range of wavelengths as do fish!

Let us look more closely at the structure of light. If we could stop a wave of light for an instant, it would look something like Figure 8.1. The

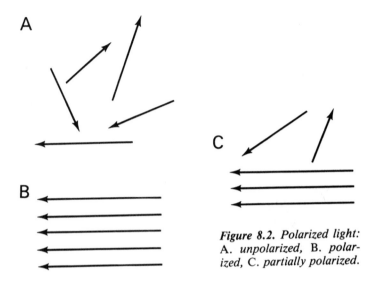

Figure 8.2. Polarized light: A. unpolarized, B. polarized, C. partially polarized.

wave is moving in the direction of the arrowhead, and perpendicular to it are the planes of the electric and magnetic fields. (The magnetic field is of no consequence for our purposes and can be ignored.) The direction of the electric field is important, for upon it depends the phenomenon of *polarization.* Figure 8.2 shows an end-on view of the electric fields in a beam of light.

The light in Figure 8.2*A* is unpolarized. All of the waves of light are coming toward the observer (out of the plane of the paper), but the directions of the electric fields are random. In comparison, Figure 8.2*B* represents polarized light, and Figure 8.2*C* partially polarized light.

Polarized and partially polarized light are produced in a number of circumstances. When sunlight is reflected from a regular surface such as water, it may be completely or partially polarized depending on the angle at which the light strikes the water; that is, the surface of the water acts to rearrange the electric fields of the light. For most surfaces, such as water or glass, the light becomes horizontally polarized as in Figure 8.2*B*.

GLARE

While sailing, we are never confronted with completely polarized light because the reflecting surface is never perfectly smooth. But enough of the sunlight is polarized to interfere with the identification of distant objects. Before we consider how polarized light impedes visual discrimination, let us look at the larger problem of *glare*. The term *glare* is used to describe the effect of excessive light. This excessive light enters the eye and tends to wash out the contrast of what we are looking at, making it difficult or impossible to identify fine detail. Everyone is familiar with the need to pull down the shade when viewing a projected slide or a television screen. In fact, during periods of glare, the eyes are receiving 10 to 100 times the amount of light they need to function optimally. Sometimes glare is the result of intense sunlight solely, but often light reflected from surfaces such as water makes a major contribution.

There are a number of practical responses to glare that interferes with vision. First, the pupils of the eyes constrict, automatically and almost instantaneously. Unfortunately, this response is not very effective. Even when the pupils are reduced to a tiny dot, they cannot eliminate much of the excess light. The next response is to eliminate some of the light physically by squinting. But there are problems with squinting; it, too, is rather ineffectual, and if the sailor squints for a prolonged period of time, he is likely to develop a headache. Rather than squinting, the sailor should wear a broad-rimmed hat or a visor. Of course, the most effective mechanism is to filter out some of the unnecessary light with sunglasses.

SUNGLASSES

All sunglasses operate by filtering out or reflecting away a certain percentage of the light rays that were otherwise destined to reach the eye. They accomplish this in one of four ways.

Neutral lenses are always various shades of gray because they filter out a certain percentage of all light rays that reach them. The darker the gray, the less light transmitted. For example, a lens that has a transmission of 20 percent filters out 80 percent of the light, i.e., 8 of every 10 light rays that strike the glass do not reach the eye. Note that neutral sunglasses affect all portions of the light spectrum equally—just as much blue is filtered as is green or red. Because of this, there is no color distortion, an important characteristic for sailors.

Colored, or *tinted, lenses* selectively affect the transmission of certain portions of the light spectrum more than others. Green sunglasses, for example, appear green because more of the green and less of the rest of the spectrum is transmitted. The overall transmission may be the same (e.g., 20 percent) as neutral lenses. It should be noted that, contrary to popular myth, yellow or amber lenses are *not* able to improve vision in either haze or fog!

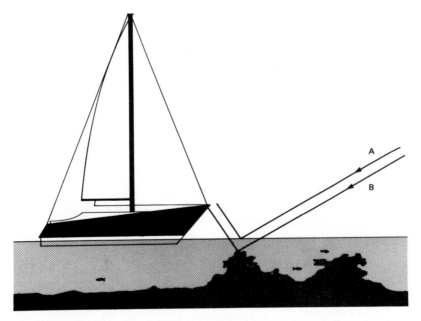

Figure 8.3. *Boat approaching a coral reef in glare. Polarized sunglasses can eliminate light ray A, which is polarized horizontally. Without light ray A, light ray B reflecting off of the coral is visible.*

Reflecting, or *mirror, lenses* act like partially silvered mirrors and reflect light away from the eye. Like neutral lenses, they represent color accurately. They are generally a very effective means of decreasing glare.

Polarizing lenses are very discriminating in their appetite for light rays. The polarizing material consists of a plastic film that has been stretched in one direction to align the individual molecules and then treated with an iodine solution. The film absorbs any light with an electric field parallel to the stretch direction. Nearly all polarized glasses are oriented horizontally to block the horizontally polarized light. In practice, some of the light polarized in other directions is also absorbed, producing a further reduction in glare.

In certain circumstances—when avoiding coral reefs, for example—the difference between sunglasses and polarized glasses can be crucial. Figure 8.3 illustrates a boat approaching a coral reef. Because of the glare from light reflected from the surface (*A*), the ability of the eye to perceive light reflected from the reef (*B*) is diminished. Ordinary sunglasses would be of little value since they would diminish both light rays. Polarized glasses, however, would preferentially eliminate light ray *A* since it most likely would be polarized horizontally. This would allow *B* to be better appreciated. Frequently the effect is dramatic—like possessing X-ray vision! Of course, this effect would not occur unless light ray *B* were transmissible; that is, the water would need to be clear and relatively free of particulate matter and surface disturbance that would scatter light ray *B* before it could reach the eye. Also, excessive light would have to be available so that we could discard some of it and still have enough left over to stimulate the eye. Polarized lenses would in no way augment the transmission of light ray *B* from the reef. Rather, they would reduce the glare from the polarized light ray *A*. In places that are "reef-strewn," such as the Caribbean, polarized glasses are invaluable.

What kind of glasses should the sailor purchase? That depends on whether or not a prescription is necessary. If not, a wide variety of plastic and glass lenses are available, including neutral or tinted lenses, photochromatic lenses (see discussion next), polarized lenses, and reflecting lenses. Any of these should be adequate for normal use provided they are dark enough. One way to tell is to put them on indoors during the day and look in a mirror. If you can see your eyes, they probably are not dark enough to offer adequate protection on the water. The choice between plastic or glass depends on the relative importance of weight versus ruggedness. Plastic is about 25 percent lighter, but it scratches more easily. If weight is the major consideration, choose plastic. However, if you tend to be rough on your glasses, scratch-resistant glass is a better bet. All glass should be of the safety (tempered) variety to decrease danger to the eye in case of cracking or breakage.

Most prescriptions are now available in sunglasses. Some of the more popular glasses include the following.

Photochromatic lenses darken on exposure to sunlight and lighten up again in the dark, thus making two pairs of eyeglasses (one for the sun and one for regular use) unnecessary. However, a few drawbacks should be kept in mind. First, they are presently available only in glass, although plastic lenses may soon be marketed. Second, the degree of both the darkening and lightening is limited. For example, Photogray Extra (Corning) darkens to 22 percent transmittance and lightens to 87 percent. Although a transmittance of 22 percent is adequate for people who spend some time outdoors, many sailors may feel more comfortable with darker lenses. In addition, there is always a slight tint in the lens. During twilight and at night, the lack of clear transmission may represent an additional, albeit minor, impediment to vision. Third, there is a time delay involved before the lenses darken and fade, which may present a problem if it becomes necessary to go below to consult a chart.

Neutral or *tinted prescription lenses* have the advantage that they can be made precisely as dark as is desired. Usually a transmission of 10 to 15 percent is the practical limit. For sailors who normally require bifocals, a gradient tint may be the answer. The upper segment for distant vision is darkened to reduce glare, whereas the lower, reading segment is clear for chart consultation.

Clip-on lenses are still preferred by some sailors. Although they add weight to the glasses, they have the distinct advantage that when covered with spray they can be removed and cleaned without losing the visual correction!

Polarized lenses and *reflecting (mirror) lenses* are both available in prescription form. In fact, probably the single, best sunglasses for sailors would be a 20 percent transmission gray lens *with* polarization added. The only drawback is that adding polarization is somewhat expensive (perhaps another 50 dollars).

Remember, caveat emptor! There are wide variations in both price and quality.

What about contact lenses at sea? Some sailors swear by them since they don't fog up or become streaked with spray or rain. The only real problem with contact lenses at sea (aside from the need to bring along additional paraphernalia) is the increased risk of corneal abrasion and ulceration. The constant wind at sea has a tendency to dry out the eyes. If the tear film, on which all contact lenses rest, should evaporate, the eye is at increased risk. *If you wear contact lenses, you must still wear some kind of glasses to lessen tear evaporation due to the wind.* Sunglasses are fine if it is bright, but for overcast days or nighttime sailing, a pair of clear glasses should be purchased. The contact lens wearer must remember to avoid *overwear* due to long watches or irregular schedules. If anything, wearing time tends to be shorter than normal. The sailor should also purchase lubricating drops (artificial tears) in case of miscalculation.

Finally, all sailors, whether they are planning to wear contact lenses or glasses, should bring along an extra pair of glasses. And the sailor should, without fail, wear a safety band with his glasses. If he doesn't, he deserves to lose them overboard!

BENDING LIGHT RAYS

As sailors we spend our time at the interface of two very different fluids, sailing through one by harnessing the power of the other. In addition to

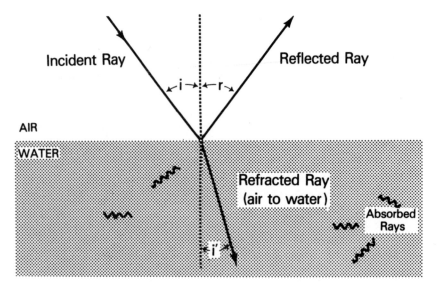

Figure 8.4. Light traveling from air to water: reflection, refraction, and absorption.

its own properties, each fluid has a third set of properties that exists only at the interface. Likewise, light behaves differently at the interface than it does in either air or water.

The speed of light is approximately 3×10^8 meters per second. But this value is strictly true only for a vacuum. As soon as light enters the atmosphere, it slows down. The velocity of all electromagnetic radiation depends on the density of the medium through which it travels: the denser the medium, the slower the travel speed. One measure of the density of the medium is the index of refraction. The higher the index of refraction, the slower the light travels. The index of refraction of water, for example, is 1.333, so that light travels only 75 percent as fast in water as it does in air.

When light strikes a surface such as water, it may be *absorbed, reflected,* or *refracted* (Figure 8.4). The amount of light that the water absorbs (and converts to heat) depends on the angle of incidence, which is greater when the sun is at the zenith than near the horizon. The degree of reflection varies with the smoothness of the surface. It is easy to see a reflection on a still lake but quite another matter on a wind-swept bay. Other rays enter the water and are bent, or refracted.[2] Usually when light strikes the water at an angle, reflection and refraction occur simultaneously; some light rays are reflected, some refracted. The properties of the surface, especially its smoothness, determine the proportion.

So far we have been concerned only with light passing from air into water, but in order to see an underwater object, this light must be reflected

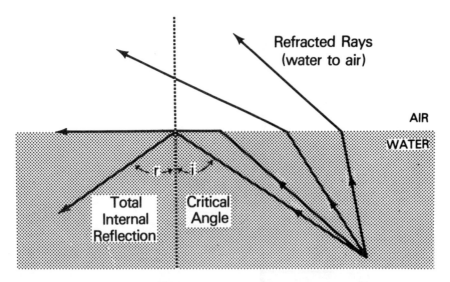

Figure 8.5. Light traveling from water to air: reflection, refraction (and absorption). Notice that if a reflected ray strikes the surface at or above a critical angle, there is total internal reflection. For this reason, the sun should be high in the sky when watching for subsurface impedimenta such as coral heads.

off of the object and traverse the surface a second time before reaching our eyes. During this second transit, light again is either absorbed, reflected, or refracted. If the light strikes the surface at too great an angle, however, it will not emerge from the water, a phenomenon called *total internal reflection* (Figure 8.5).

If the light does escape the surface, our eyes and brain can never discern its precise origin. *All that we can perceive is the direction from which light strikes the retina of the eye.* After all, when we see ourselves reflected in a still lake or a mirror, it appears that we are *in* the water or *behind* the mirror because the light is coming from that direction. In other words, we note the direction from which the light arrives and *assume* that since light usually travels in a straight line the object must be at the end of that straight line. Figure 8.6 illustrates this illusion. Due to refraction, an underwater object appears shallower and larger than it really is. This concept of *image displacement* is crucial to understanding all of the maritime optical illusions that are discussed in this chapter.

LIGHT AND THE UPPER ATMOSPHERE

Now let us consider how the atmosphere itself affects light. The atmosphere

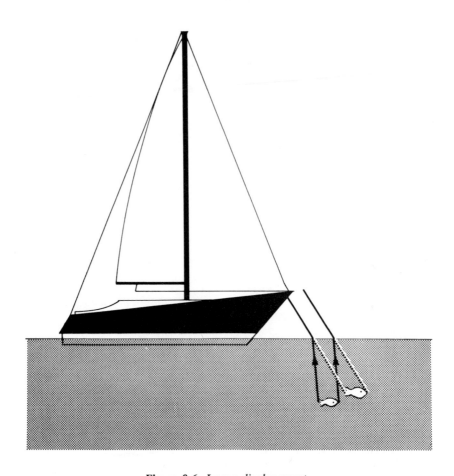

Figure 8.6. *Image displacement.*

is responsible for such diverse phenomena as blue skies, red sunsets, the "green flash," and marine mirages.

If we pause to consider the propagation of light, it seems paradoxical that we routinely perceive light from stars billions of miles away, yet, at the same time, strain to see a buoy light at a scant distance of 1 mile. The reason is that interstellar space is so rarefied that there is almost nothing to impede the progress of light rays until they enter our atmosphere. Once within the atmosphere, they run an increasing risk of colliding with one or more of the atmospheric molecules.

Imagine a shaft of light piercing a dusty room. As light strikes a dust particle, it is radiated in all directions—so-called *light scatter*. We see the shaft of light because of the sideways scatter from each dust particle. If the room were perfectly free of dust, the shaft of light would be invisible. A similar scattering occurs when light from the sun strikes the air molecules

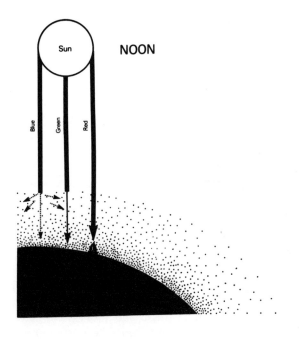

NOON

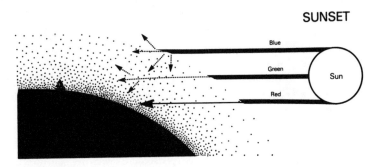

SUNSET

Figure 8.7. The appearance of the sun and sky at both noon and sunset. At noon the blue wavelengths are scattered throughout the sky, while the sun appears yellow from the mixture of red and green wavelengths. At sunset progressively longer wavelengths become scattered, producing a red sun and a multicolored sunset.

of the atmosphere. This is known as Rayleigh scatter, after Lord Rayleigh, who showed that the shorter blue wavelengths are scattered much more than the longer green and red wavelengths. The blue appearance of the sky is due to the fact that blue is scattered 16 times as much as red! At noon, when the sun is high in the sky, the sunlight strikes the atmosphere in an almost perpendicular fashion and blue light is scattered over the sky (Figure 8.7). These rays are eventually scattered down to earth. The scat-

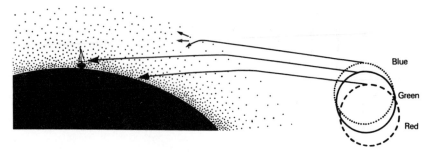

Figure 8.8. The green flash.

tering removes some of the blue color from the appearance of the sun, leaving the red and the green, which together produce its yellowish hue.[3] As the sun continues to approach the horizon, the light rays strike the atmosphere at an increasingly larger angle and must travel a greater distance through the atmosphere. As the distance increases, the longer wavelengths of green now begin to be scattered. The additional scatter of green means that the light rays that reach the earth are a mixture of oranges and reds. These colors are prominent low in the western sky at sunset, while the blues and purples predominate higher. The play of these colors upon the clouds and atmospheric contaminants creates the spectacle of sunset. The sun itself, progressively stripped of its longer wavelengths as it nears the horizon, undergoes its own variegated metamorphosis from yellow to orange to red.

If conditions are favorable, and if the sailor is attentive, he may be treated to an unusual, albeit brief, phenomenon—the *green flash.* As light passes through the atmosphere, it is refracted as well as scattered. The amount of refraction is slightly different for each wavelength. As a result, multiple images of the sun occur, each of a different color—a kind of prismatic spectrum of images (Figure 8.8). The difference in "register" between the images is usually imperceptible except near the horizon, where the prismatic dispersion between the blue and red images may amount to 10 seconds of arc. The red light refracts the least so that the red disk is the first to set. The atmosphere scatters most of the blue light. Thus, as the sun sets, there may be a brief period when the green image is the only one visible. It is called the green flash because not only does the upper rim appear green, but green rays seem to emanate from this upper rim. The green flash usually lasts only 1 to 2 seconds, and conditions must be favorable to see it at all. There must be a sharp horizon, good visibility, preferably a temperature inversion, and, most important, an attentive observer. It is difficult to achieve these conditions anywhere *except* at sea, which is why the green flash is fundamentally a marine phenomenon. In polar regions, because of tremendous refraction, the green flash may last for 15 minutes. The record sighting seems to belong to Admiral Richard Byrd. During his expedition to the South Pole in 1929, he witnessed the green flash intermittently at sunset for 35 minutes! (One caveat: It is impossible to photograph the green flash without special equipment.)

REFRACTION AND NAVIGATION

Consider this: With rare exception, every object that we see in the sky, whether it be sun, moon, planet, or star, is not where it appears to be! Refraction displaces the image of these objects in the celestial vault except when they are precisely overhead at the zenith. Even at the zenith, some refractive bending may occur if the various layers of the atmosphere are tilted slightly one to another.

If it is true that no celestial object is where it appears to be, how are our celestial measurements ever accurate? The answer is that scientists have conducted a considerable amount of research to determine the precise amount of refraction at each altitude. The values are contained in Tables 8.1 and 8.2, reprinted from the *Nautical Almanac*.[4] Table 8.1 covers altitudes 10 to 90 degrees, whereas Table 8.2 contains the low-altitude calculations, 0 to 10 degrees.

In order to appreciate the degree of astronomic refraction, we need only peruse the columns headed "Stars and Planets." Stars (as well as planets most of the time) are so distant that they can be considered as point sources of light. A point source has no significant diameter. The mean diameter of the sun and moon, however, are both about 32 minutes of arc and cannot be so neglected. The *Nautical Almanac* combines the correction for semidiameter with the correction for refraction and presents a single correction. Since the stars are point sources of light, the values in Tables 8.1 and 8.2 represent the *pure* refractive power of the atmosphere for each particular altitude.

We predicted that at the zenith there would be no refraction, and indeed from an apparent altitude of 90 degrees to 87 degrees 3 minutes, there is no correction. (If we examine the sun columns at the zenith, the correction factor, depending on the season, is either 15.9 minutes or 16.2 minutes, which is the semidiameter of the sun. In fact, if 16 minutes are subtracted from any sun correction, the remaining value is the refraction component and is approximately equal to the star correction.)

TABLE 8.1*
Altitude Correction Tables, 10°–90°

Source: Table A2, The Nautical Almanac.

SUN

OCT.–MAR. App. Alt.	Lower Limb	Upper Limb	APR.–SEPT. App. Alt.	Lower Limb	Upper Limb
9 34	+10.8	−21.5	9 39	+10.6	−21.2
9 45	+10.9	−21.4	9 51	+10.7	−21.1
9 56	+11.0	−21.3	10 03	+10.8	−21.0
10 08	+11.1	−21.2	10 15	+10.9	−20.9
10 21	+11.2	−21.1	10 27	+11.0	−20.8
10 34	+11.3	−21.0	10 40	+11.1	−20.7
10 47	+11.4	−20.9	10 54	+11.2	−20.6
11 01	+11.5	−20.8	11 08	+11.3	−20.5
11 15	+11.6	−20.7	11 23	+11.4	−20.4
11 30	+11.7	−20.6	11 38	+11.5	−20.3
11 46	+11.8	−20.5	11 54	+11.6	−20.2
12 02	+11.9	−20.4	12 10	+11.7	−20.1
12 19	+12.0	−20.3	12 28	+11.8	−20.0
12 37	+12.1	−20.2	12 46	+11.9	−19.9
12 55	+12.2	−20.1	13 05	+12.0	−19.8
13 14	+12.3	−20.0	13 24	+12.1	−19.7
13 35	+12.4	−19.9	13 45	+12.2	−19.6
13 56	+12.5	−19.8	14 07	+12.3	−19.5
14 18	+12.6	−19.7	14 30	+12.4	−19.4
14 42	+12.7	−19.6	14 54	+12.5	−19.3
15 06	+12.8	−19.5	15 19	+12.6	−19.2
15 32	+12.9	−19.4	15 46	+12.7	−19.1
15 59	+13.0	−19.3	16 14	+12.8	−19.0
16 28	+13.1	−19.2	16 44	+12.9	−18.9
16 59	+13.2	−19.1	17 15	+13.0	−18.8
17 32	+13.3	−19.0	17 48	+13.1	−18.7
18 06	+13.4	−18.9	18 24	+13.2	−18.6
18 42	+13.5	−18.8	19 01	+13.3	−18.5
19 21	+13.6	−18.7	19 42	+13.4	−18.4
20 03	+13.7	−18.6	20 25	+13.5	−18.3
20 48	+13.8	−18.5	21 11	+13.6	−18.2
21 35	+13.9	−18.4	22 00	+13.7	−18.1
22 26	+14.0	−18.3	22 54	+13.8	−18.0
23 22	+14.1	−18.2	23 51	+13.9	−17.9
24 21	+14.2	−18.1	24 53	+14.0	−17.8
25 26	+14.3	−18.0	26 00	+14.1	−17.7
26 36	+14.4	−17.9	27 13	+14.2	−17.6
27 52	+14.5	−17.8	28 33	+14.3	−17.5
29 15	+14.6	−17.7	30 00	+14.4	−17.4
30 46	+14.7	−17.6	31 35	+14.5	−17.3
32 26	+14.8	−17.5	33 20	+14.6	−17.2
34 17	+14.9	−17.4	35 17	+14.7	−17.1
36 20	+15.0	−17.3	37 26	+14.8	−17.0
38 36	+15.1	−17.2	39 50	+14.9	−16.9
41 08	+15.2	−17.1	42 31	+15.0	−16.8
43 59	+15.3	−17.0	45 31	+15.1	−16.7
47 10	+15.4	−16.9	48 55	+15.2	−16.6
50 46	+15.5	−16.8	52 44	+15.3	−16.5
54 49	+15.6	−16.7	57 02	+15.4	−16.4
59 23	+15.7	−16.6	61 51	+15.5	−16.3
64 30	+15.8	−16.5	67 17	+15.6	−16.2
70 12	+15.9	−16.4	73 16	+15.7	−16.1
76 26	+16.0	−16.3	79 43	+15.8	−16.0
83 05	+16.1	−16.2	86 32	+15.9	−15.9
90 00			90 00		

STARS AND PLANETS

App. Alt.	Corrn	App. Alt.	Additional Corrn
9 56	−5.3		**1983**
10 08	−5.2		**VENUS**
10 20	−5.1		Jan. 1–May 10
10 33	−5.0		42° + 0.1
10 46	−4.9		
11 00	−4.8		May 11–June 23
11 14	−4.7		47° + 0.2
11 29	−4.6		
11 45	−4.5		June 24–July 19
12 01	−4.4		46° + 0.3
12 18	−4.3		
12 35	−4.2		July 20–Aug. 3
12 54	−4.1		11° + 0.4
13 13	−4.0		41° + 0.5
13 33	−3.9		
13 54	−3.8		Aug. 4–Aug. 12
14 16	−3.7		6° + 0.5
14 40	−3.6		20° + 0.6
15 04	−3.5		31° + 0.7
15 30	−3.4		
15 57	−3.3		Aug. 13–Sept. 7
16 26	−3.2		4° + 0.6
16 56	−3.1		12° + 0.7
17 28	−3.0		22° + 0.8
18 02	−2.9		
18 38	−2.8		
19 17	−2.7		Sept. 8–Sept. 16
19 58	−2.6		6° + 0.5
20 42	−2.5		20° + 0.6
21 28	−2.4		31° + 0.7
22 19	−2.3		
23 13	−2.2		Sept. 17–Oct. 2
24 11	−2.1		11° + 0.4
25 14	−2.0		41° + 0.5
26 22	−1.9		
27 36	−1.8		Oct. 3–Oct. 30
28 56	−1.7		46° + 0.3
30 24	−1.6		
32 00	−1.5		Oct. 31–Dec. 17
33 45	−1.4		47° + 0.2
35 40	−1.3		
37 48	−1.2		Dec. 18–Dec. 31
40 08	−1.1		42° + 0.1
42 44	−1.0		
45 36	−0.9		
48 47	−0.8		
52 18	−0.7		**MARS**
56 11	−0.6		Jan. 1–Dec. 31
60 28	−0.5		60° + 0.1
65 08	−0.4		
70 11	−0.3		
75 34	−0.2		
81 13	−0.1		
87 03	0.0		
90 00			

DIP

Ht. of Eye (m)	Corrn	Ht. of Eye (ft)	Ht. of Eye	Corrn
2.4	−2.8	8.0	m	
2.6	−2.9	8.6	1.0 − 1.8	
2.8	−3.0	9.2	1.5 − 2.2	
3.0	−3.1	9.8	2.0 − 2.5	
3.2	−3.2	10.5	2.5 − 2.8	
3.4	−3.3	11.2	3.0 − 3.0	
3.6	−3.4	11.9	See table ←	
3.8	−3.5	12.6		
4.0	−3.6	13.3	m	
4.3	−3.7	14.1	20 − 7.9	
4.5	−3.8	14.9	22 − 8.3	
4.7	−3.9	15.7	24 − 8.6	
5.0	−4.0	16.5	26 − 9.0	
5.2	−4.1	17.4	28 − 9.3	
5.5	−4.2	18.3		
5.8	−4.3	19.1	30 − 9.6	
6.1	−4.4	20.1	32 − 10.0	
6.3	−4.5	21.0	34 − 10.3	
6.6	−4.6	22.0	36 − 10.6	
6.9	−4.7	22.9	38 − 10.8	
7.2	−4.8	23.9		
7.5	−4.9	24.9	40 − 11.1	
7.9	−5.0	26.0	42 − 11.4	
8.2	−5.1	27.1	44 − 11.7	
8.5	−5.2	28.1	46 − 11.9	
8.8	−5.3	29.2	48 − 12.2	
9.2	−5.4	30.4	ft.	
9.5	−5.5	31.5	2 − 1.4	
9.9	−5.6	32.7	4 − 1.9	
10.3	−5.7	33.9	6 − 2.4	
10.6	−5.8	35.1	8 − 2.7	
11.0	−5.9	36.3	10 − 3.1	
11.4	−6.0	37.6	See table ←	
11.8	−6.1	38.9	ft.	
12.2	−6.2	40.1	70 − 8.1	
12.6	−6.3	41.5	75 − 8.4	
13.0	−6.4	42.8	80 − 8.7	
13.4	−6.5	44.2	85 − 8.9	
13.8	−6.6	45.5	90 − 9.2	
14.2	−6.7	46.9	95 − 9.5	
14.7	−6.8	48.4	100 − 9.7	
15.1	−6.9	49.8	105 − 9.9	
15.5	−7.0	51.3	110 − 10.2	
16.0	−7.1	52.8	115 − 10.4	
16.5	−7.2	54.3	120 − 10.6	
16.9	−7.3	55.8	125 − 10.8	
17.4	−7.4	57.4		
17.9	−7.5	58.9	130 − 11.1	
18.4	−7.6	60.5	135 − 11.3	
18.8	−7.7	62.1	140 − 11.5	
19.3	−7.8	63.8	145 − 11.7	
19.8	−7.9	65.4	150 − 11.9	
20.4	−8.0	67.1	155 − 12.1	
20.9	−8.1	68.8		
21.4		70.5		

TABLE 8.2*
Altitude Correction Tables, 0°–10°

App. Alt.	OCT.–MAR. SUN Lower Limb	Upper Limb	APR.–SEPT. Lower Limb	Upper Limb	STARS PLANETS
0 00	−18.2	−50.5	−18.4	−50.2	−34.5
03	17.5	49.8	17.8	49.6	33.8
06	16.9	49.2	17.1	48.9	33.2
09	16.3	48.6	16.5	48.3	32.6
12	15.7	48.0	15.9	47.7	32.0
15	15.1	47.4	15.3	47.1	31.4
0 18	−14.5	−46.8	−14.8	−46.6	−30.8
21	14.0	46.3	14.2	46.0	30.3
24	13.5	45.8	13.7	45.5	29.8
27	12.9	45.2	13.2	45.0	29.2
30	12.4	44.7	12.7	44.5	28.7
33	11.9	44.2	12.2	44.0	28.2
0 36	−11.5	−43.8	−11.7	−43.5	−27.8
39	11.0	43.3	11.2	43.0	27.3
42	10.5	42.8	10.8	42.6	26.8
45	10.1	42.4	10.3	42.1	26.4
48	9.6	41.9	9.9	41.7	25.9
51	9.2	41.5	9.5	41.3	25.5
0 54	−8.8	−41.1	−9.1	−40.9	−25.1
0 57	8.4	40.7	8.7	40.5	24.7
1 00	8.0	40.3	8.3	40.1	24.3
03	7.7	40.0	7.9	39.7	24.0
06	7.3	39.6	7.5	39.3	23.6
09	6.9	39.2	7.2	39.0	23.2
1 12	−6.6	−38.9	−6.8	−38.6	−22.9
15	6.2	38.5	6.5	38.3	22.5
18	5.9	38.2	6.2	38.0	22.2
21	5.6	37.9	5.8	37.6	21.9
24	5.3	37.6	5.5	37.3	21.6
27	4.9	37.2	5.2	37.0	21.2
1 30	−4.6	−36.9	−4.9	−36.7	−20.9
35	4.2	36.5	4.4	36.2	20.5
40	3.7	36.0	4.0	35.8	20.0
45	3.2	35.5	3.5	35.3	19.5
50	2.8	35.1	3.1	34.9	19.1
1 55	2.4	34.7	2.6	34.4	18.7
2 00	−2.0	−34.3	−2.2	−34.0	−18.3
05	1.6	33.9	1.8	33.6	17.9
10	1.2	33.5	1.5	33.3	17.5
15	0.9	33.2	1.1	32.9	17.2
20	0.5	32.8	0.8	32.6	16.8
25	−0.2	32.5	0.4	32.2	16.5
2 30	+0.2	−32.1	−0.1	−31.9	−16.1
35	0.5	31.8	+0.2	31.6	15.8
40	0.8	31.5	0.5	31.3	15.5
45	1.1	31.2	0.8	31.0	15.2
50	1.4	30.9	1.1	30.7	14.9
2 55	1.6	30.7	1.4	30.4	14.7
3 00	+1.9	−30.4	+1.7	−30.1	−14.4
05	2.2	30.1	1.9	29.9	14.1
10	2.4	29.9	2.1	29.7	13.9
15	2.6	29.7	2.4	29.4	13.7
20	2.9	29.4	2.6	29.2	13.4
25	3.1	29.2	2.9	28.9	13.2
3 30	+3.3	−29.0	+3.1	−28.7	−13.0

App. Alt.	OCT.–MAR. SUN Lower Limb	Upper Limb	APR.–SEPT. Lower Limb	Upper Limb	STARS PLANETS
3 30	+3.3	−29.0	+3.1	−28.7	−13.0
35	3.6	28.7	3.3	28.5	12.7
40	3.8	28.5	3.5	28.3	12.5
45	4.0	28.3	3.7	28.1	12.3
50	4.2	28.1	3.9	27.9	12.1
3 55	4.4	27.9	4.1	27.7	11.9
4 00	+4.5	−27.8	+4.3	−27.5	−11.8
05	4.7	27.6	4.5	27.3	11.6
10	4.9	27.4	4.6	27.2	11.4
15	5.1	27.2	4.8	27.0	11.2
20	5.2	27.1	5.0	26.8	11.1
25	5.4	26.9	5.1	26.7	10.9
4 30	+5.6	−26.7	+5.3	−26.5	−10.7
35	5.7	26.6	5.5	26.3	10.6
40	5.9	26.4	5.6	26.2	10.4
45	6.0	26.3	5.8	26.0	10.3
50	6.2	26.1	5.9	25.9	10.1
4 55	6.3	26.0	6.0	25.8	10.0
5 00	+6.4	−25.9	+6.2	−25.6	−9.9
05	6.6	25.7	6.3	25.5	9.7
10	6.7	25.6	6.4	25.4	9.6
15	6.8	25.5	6.6	25.2	9.5
20	6.9	25.4	6.7	25.1	9.4
25	7.1	25.2	6.8	25.0	9.2
5 30	+7.2	−25.1	+6.9	−24.9	−9.1
35	7.3	25.0	7.0	24.8	9.0
40	7.4	24.9	7.2	24.6	8.9
45	7.5	24.8	7.3	24.5	8.8
50	7.6	24.7	7.4	24.4	8.7
5 55	7.7	24.6	7.5	24.3	8.6
6 00	+7.8	−24.5	+7.6	−24.2	−8.5
10	8.0	24.3	7.8	24.0	8.3
20	8.2	24.1	8.0	23.8	8.1
30	8.4	23.9	8.1	23.7	7.9
40	8.6	23.7	8.3	23.5	7.7
6 50	8.7	23.6	8.5	23.3	7.6
7 00	+8.9	−23.4	+8.6	−23.2	−7.4
10	9.1	23.2	8.8	23.0	7.2
20	9.2	23.1	9.0	22.8	7.1
30	9.3	23.0	9.1	22.7	7.0
40	9.5	22.8	9.2	22.6	6.8
7 50	9.6	22.7	9.4	22.4	6.7
8 00	+9.7	−22.6	+9.5	−22.3	−6.6
10	9.9	22.4	9.6	22.2	6.4
20	10.0	22.3	9.7	22.1	6.3
30	10.1	22.2	9.8	22.0	6.2
40	10.2	22.1	10.0	21.8	6.1
8 50	10.3	22.0	10.1	21.7	6.0
9 00	+10.4	−21.9	+10.2	−21.6	−5.9
10	10.5	21.8	10.3	21.5	5.8
20	10.6	21.7	10.4	21.4	5.7
30	10.7	21.6	10.5	21.3	5.6
40	10.8	21.5	10.6	21.2	5.5
9 50	10.9	21.4	10.6	21.2	5.4
10 00	+11.0	−21.3	+10.7	−21.1	−5.3

*Source: Table A3, The Nautical Almanac.

As the star begins to descend in altitude, the degree of refraction is at first quite modest (Table 8.1). At an altitude of 40 degrees, it is about 1.2 minutes; at 20 degrees, 2.6 minutes; at 10 degrees, 5.3 minutes. Thenceforth, as the star nears the horizon, the magnitude of the refraction increases rapidly (Table 8.2). At 5 degrees, it is 9.9 minutes; at 2 degrees, 18.3 minutes; and at 0 degree, 34.5 minutes. The values for stars and planets are always *negative* because refraction causes a celestial body to appear *higher* than it is.

Since the mean diameter of the sun and moon are about 32 minutes of arc and since the refraction at 0 degree altitude is 34.5 minutes of arc, when the lower limb of either body is just tangent to the horizon, the entire sun or moon is actually below the horizon. This is certainly an extreme example of a celestial body not being where it appears to be!

Because refraction is a major source of error in celestial observation, particularly of objects at low altitudes, navigators in the past have generally eschewed low-altitude observations. The lower limit has been considered to be 15 degrees. Although it remains good nautical practice to choose high-altitude objects if they are available, objects as low as 5 degrees can now be employed with confidence. Sights lower than that should be treated with caution, although, if atmospheric conditions are not extreme, even they provide usable information.

The values in Tables 8.1 and 8.2 represent average values or *mean refraction*. The values are based upon a surface air temperature of 50° F (10° C) and an atmospheric pressure of 29.83 inches (1,010 millibars) of mercury. Although they take into account the effects of astronomic refraction, terrestrial refraction—due to temperature and pressure variations near the surface—is ignored. The *Nautical Almanac* provides an additional table to correct for these variations. In practice this table is rarely used unless the atmospheric conditions are rather extreme or the altitude of the object is low in the sky. However frequently terrestrial refraction is ignored in the routine practice of navigation, the surface atmospheric conditions that cause it are capable of effecting the most phenomenal spectacles.

TERRESTRIAL REFRACTION AND "FLYAWAY ISLANDS"

In 1906, during one of his attempts to reach the North Pole, Robert E. Peary stood at the summit of Cape Thomas Hubbard. About 120 miles (194 kilometers) to the northwest he saw "snow-clad summits above the ice horizon." Later he again saw the spectacular land in the distance and christened it Crocker Land. He wrote, "My heart leaped the intervening miles of ice as I looked longingly at this land and, in fancy, I trod its shores and climbed its summits, even though I knew that that pleasure could be only for another in another season."[5]

Donald B. MacMillan was destined to lead the expedition to Crocker Land. His party set forth in 1913, but it was not until the following year that they were able to reach Cape Thomas Hubbard. Despite temperatures as low as $-25°$ F ($-32°$ C) and dangerously thin ice, the expedition traveled northwest for several days. MacMillan wrote in his diary, "This morning...Crocker Land was in sight. We all rushed out and up to the top of a berg. Sure enough! There it was as plain as day—hills, valleys, and ice cap, a tremendous land extending through 150 degrees of the horizon."[6] The expedition party then traveled more than 130 miles (210 kilometers) over the polar sea far beyond the place where Crocker Land was seen. Yet there was nothing. Crocker Land was a mirage!

In addition to tantalizing polar explorers, these visual illusions may have indirectly acted as an impetus to the discovery of the New World. But these illusions have more than historic interest for the modern sailor. They have the potential to influence visual piloting and navigation, in either a positive or a negative fashion, and like the green flash, these wonderful phenomena are particularly frequent at sea.

All of the visual illusions now under consideration are due to *terrestrial refraction*. Astronomic refraction, as we have seen, produces its effects at the higher reaches of our atmosphere. Since the upper atmosphere is relatively unchanging, the visual illusions due to astronomic refraction are quite predictable; witness Tables 8.1 and 8.2. Terrestrial refraction is a phenomenon of the lower atmosphere—from the surface to perhaps 1,000 feet (300 meters) at most. As we are well aware, this portion of the atmosphere is in a rapid state of flux and accounts for the unpredictability and evanescence of all of these spectacles.

In order to understand what creates the illusions, we need to consider a few basic concepts of surface meteorology:

1. The index of refraction of air (the average value for which is 1.0003) varies with air density. The density in turn is dependent on three factors: temperature, pressure, and humidity. In reality neither pressure nor humidity exerts an appreciable effect, so we can pretend that the air density, and hence the index of refraction, varies with temperature. A high temperature produces a low density and a low index of refraction. Low temperature, conversely, corresponds to high density and a high index of refraction. The greater the *density gradient* (the change of density with height), the greater the *index of refraction gradient* and the greater the refractive bending of light rays.

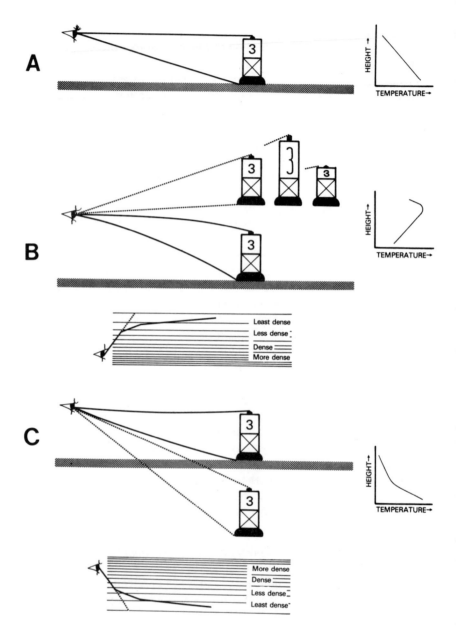

Figure 8.9. *Normal vision at sea* (A); *looming, with towering and stooping* (B); *sinking* (C).

2. Air generally becomes less dense with increasing height above the surface of the earth.

3. Temperature normally decreases with increasing height above the surface; air is colder aloft. In meteorologic parlance, the temperature-height profile is known as the lapse-rate (Figure 8.9*A*). An inverted profile with warmer air above cooler air is called a temperature inversion.

English sailors have recognized the phenomenon of *looming* at least since the 19th century, when the word officially entered the English language. These sailors realized that under certain atmospheric conditions a light or a rock or any other object might loom on the horizon before it was expected to be visible.

Looming is apt to occur in middle to high latitudes when the underlying water is cool, although it may occur anytime that warmer air settles over cooler water; that is, whenever there is a temperature inversion near the surface (Figure 8.9*B*). The temperature inversion accentuates the decrease in density that normally occurs with an increase in height (see number 2 of list) and also produces less dense air aloft than near the surface. The combination produces an abnormally large density gradient near the surface, which means that there is an abnormally large index of refraction gradient. The greater the density gradient, the greater the amount of refraction.

This index of refraction gradient causes light rays that enter it to be bent down toward the surface of the earth, in turn producing an apparent elevation of the object (object displacement). The optics of terrestrial refraction obeys the general rules of refraction; thus, as light travels from a less dense medium into a more dense medium, it is always bent toward the perpendicular to the surface. Compare, for example, Figure 8.4 and Figure 8.9*B*. Light traveling from air to water (Figure 8.4) is bent more abruptly, however, than light traveling through varying densities of air (Figure 8.9*B*). This is due to the transition in the index of refraction between air (1.0003) and water (1.333). Terrestrial refraction occurs gradually over a gradient of changing layers; the light rays are actually bent at each of these thin layers. However, the direction of the final refraction nearest the observer determines the apparent position of the object in space.

When the decrease in density is relatively uniform, the upper portion of the object is refracted about the same as the lower portion, and the size of the object is unaltered. If a nonlinear change of density with height occurs so that the uppermost rays have a greater curvature, *towering* is said to exist (Figure 8.9*B*). Conversely, if the curvature at the top is less, *stooping* occurs.

Sinking can be thought of as the opposite of looming. The image now appears displaced below the object (Figure 8.9*C*). The conditions that favor sinking are quite different from those that promote looming. As Figure 8.9*C* illustrates, there is a marked increase in the temperature gradient near the surface. The warmer surface produces a layer of heated superadjacent air that is less dense than the air aloft (the opposite of normal). In this instance, light rays are refracted up to the observer, producing an apparent depression of the object. Depending on the linearity or nonlinearity of the density gradient, towering or stooping may accompany sinking. Since the necessary prerequisite for sinking is a layer of warm air immediately above the surface, this phenomenon is not uncommon over warm, open water in the wintertime. The layer of cooler, winter air in contact with the warmer water is heated from below. Actually, this temperature profile is also quite common over any enclosed body of water in the early morning. Water retains its heat through the night much better than does the adjacent land, which cools off. Cool air from the land may then flow out over the warmer water and be heated from below.

The clarity of the image is extremely variable. At times the image is reproduced with remarkable fidelity, whereas at others it is indistinct. Generally speaking, the image sinking produces (and its first cousin the inferior mirage) is less well defined. The atmospheric conditions responsible tend to be inherently *unstable*, in contrast to the temperature inversion, which is meteorologically stable. The surface instability produces rapid fluctuations in the image known as *optical shimmer*. An everyday example of optical shimmer is the distortion of distant objects when viewed through the hot exhaust gases of a jet airplane.

Obviously both looming and sinking may respectively assist or hinder visual piloting by making the image of the object appear earlier or later than expected. Frequently the loom of an object is sufficiently defined to obtain a bearing despite the fact that the object cannot be identified.

With both looming and sinking, the refractive effect of the atmosphere has been likened to a giant atmospheric lens. Certainly it is unlike the lens of a camera or that of the eye in that its huge size defies precise measurement and its refractive properties are somewhat capricious. But the analogy is nonetheless valuable. One unusual feature of the atmospheric lens is that both the observer and the object are inside of it!

This phenomenon does not occur with the illusions known as *superior* and *inferior mirages*. These mirages are produced under atmospheric conditions that promote strong stratification of the air, unlike the more gradual stratification in the previous situations. Not only is the stratification well localized, but the observer is now outside of the lens. Figure 8.10*A*

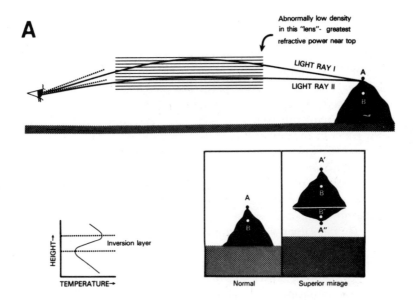

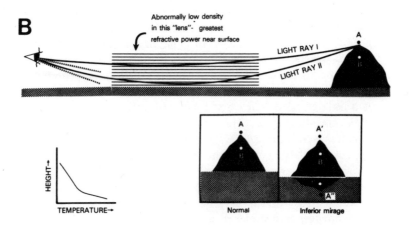

Figure 8.10. Nautical mirages: superior (A) and inferior (B).

illustrates the optics of a superior mirage. Just as in looming, there is a temperature inversion, but in this case the base of the temperature inversion is above the height of the observer—the lens is suspended in the sky. This allows light rays from the same point on the object (point *A*, for example) to travel two different pathways through the atmosphere to the observer's eye, and the observer perceives the image of this point at two widely disparate positions in space. The image nearest to the observer is nearly always the inverted one. The conditions favorable to a superior mirage are frequently found in lakes, bays, and sounds in the early afternoon. Air over the adjacent land that the sun has vigorously heated may waft over the water above the height of the observer.

An inferior mirage is illustrated in Figure 8.10*B*. The atmospheric conditions are similar to those that promote sinking, i.e., warm air near the surface, except that there is greater stratification and the lens, or superstratified layer of warm air, is immediately above the surface of the water. (In flat, desert regions the inferior mirage produces the well-known oasis illusion. A portion of the blue sky is "brought down" to earth by the tremendous refractive power of the warm air just above the desert surface.) Again, light rays may reach the observer by two different routes.

The visual illusions we have considered to this point have been distortions of a *real* distant object. But the most wondrous illusions, such as Crocker Land, result from visual distortion of the surface of the water itself. In a superior or inferior mirage, not only is the distant object distorted, but so is the horizon. In a superior mirage, the horizon is elevated (Figure 8.10*A*), creating the impression that the observer is inside of a large, flat, shallow bowl. The use of binoculars heightens this impression. Sir Francis Chichester has described this phenomenon: "Sometimes I saw strange things. Just before crossing the Line the boat appeared to be sailing up a gently sloping sea surface, in other words, uphill. At the time I was a little worried, but when I was 240 miles north of the Line I noticed the same thing again. This time the sea appeared uphill in every direction, as if I were sailing in a shallow saucer."[7] Conversely, an inferior mirage (Figure 8.10*B*) creates the sensation of being on top of a similar, but now inverted bowl—one way of feeling "on top of the world." Needless to say, if either of these conditions prevails, the *dip* correction for celestial observations may be grossly in error, overestimated with superior mirages and underestimated with inferior mirages.

If conditions are right, the sailor may experience the most enchanting illusion of all, the so-called Fata Morgana ("Fairy Morgan" in Italian). In many of the Arthurian legends, Arthur's half-sister Morgan Le Fay is credited with the ability to create magical castles in the air. Robert

Peary's Crocker Land is a typical example of a Fata Morgana. An Italian priest who witnessed a mirage over the Straits of Messina in 1643 provides an early description. While looking across the water, "the ocean which washes the coast of Sicily rose up and looked like a dark mountain range... there quickly appeared a series of more than 10,000 pilasters which were a whitish-gray color... [then the] pilasters shrank to half their height and built arches like those of Roman aqueducts."[8] The finale consisted of castles with the individual towers and windows visible.

The prerequisites for this mirage are complex, but similar to those for the superior mirage. The water at the horizon, instead of appearing to rise up slightly (producing the bowl illusion), now is markedly distorted to form a visual wall. The key to the illusion is that the brightness of the face of the wall is not uniform. Rather, it is composed of bright and dark patches irregularly elongated (towering) and shrunk (stooping), a kind of atmospheric astigmatism. The light rays from the surface of the water, which undergo vertical elongation (towering), spread their light over a greater distance and appear darker. The rays that undergo stooping are concentrated and thus look bright. The patches vary in size and shape as shimmering and gravity waves affect the atmosphere.

All that the eye perceives are these irregular, distorted, bright and dark patches. The rest the brain "imaginatively" interprets. Just as the brain constructs a Picasso nude from a single curved black line on a white background, so it formulates the most fantastic patterns from these patches of light and darkness above the horizon.

Undoubtedly men have been treated to mirages since prehistoric time. Yet there is a curious silence regarding them in historic documents. There is no reason to believe that atmospheric conditions have changed drastically in the last few thousand years. Then why are mirages not mentioned in Egyptian, biblical, or Roman sources? Probably the first mirage to be documented was the original Fata Morgana, which appears periodically off the Straits of Messina, and this was not until after the Crusades.

One plausible explanation is that although these mirages were witnessed, their insubstantiality was not appreciated; in other words, they were probably considered real! The original Fata Morgana was the first to be recognized as a mirage because the geography of the region was well known to Mediterranean sailors. They knew that there was no island there. In other regions, subjected to less maritime scrutiny than the Mediterranean, it would be difficult to disprove the ineluctability of the visual. Is there any evidence for this hypothesis?

S. E. Morison describes many "mythical" islands in *The European Discovery of America: The Northern Voyages*. These islands, located off the west coasts of Europe and Africa, were periodically sighted, but whenever they were searched for, they seemed to disappear. Sailors had a term for these illusive islands: *Flyaway Islands.* Two of the most prominent were Antilia and Hy-Brasil (or O'Brazil). Hy-Brasil is Gaelic for "isle of the blessed" and has nothing to do with the South American country. This island was regularly glimpsed from the Aran Islands and the west coast of Ireland. Its appearance on nautical charts dates back to 1325. Amazingly, it continued to appear on charts of the British Admiralty until 1873, despite the fact that shipping had traversed the area for centuries. Admiral Morison relates that "fishermen of the Aran Islands told Professor Westropp of the Royal Irish Academy that it appeared every seven years; he saw it himself in 1872! 'Just as the sun went down, a dark island suddenly appeared far out to sea, but not on the horizon. It had two hills, one wooded; between them from a low plane, rose towers and curls of smoke.' "[9]

Another mythical island that rivaled Hy-Brasil in longevity was Antilia (which means "island opposite," since it was opposite Portugal). Usually the island was charted with smaller daughter islands. Connected with this island was the recurring myth of the Seven Cities of Gold. Antilia was not "disembodied" until the 19th century. Columbus was well aware of the Antilia-Seven Cities legend. "His son states that the Discoverer wished to find 'some island' en route, as a convenient staging point for the ocean route to the Indies. And his sea journal from 25 September 1492 proves that he expected to find it about where [his chart] placed Antilia."[10] Thus the mythical island of Antilia undoubtedly contributed to Columbus's belief that a westward route to the Indies was feasible. Ironically, once news of his discovery reached Europe, skeptics disparaged the achievement by proclaiming that he had discovered nothing more than Antilia! This misconception is forever enshrined in the Portuguese and French names for the islands: As Antillas and Les Antilles.

Terrestrial refraction may have hastened the discovery of the New World in yet another way. It has been speculated that the Celtic and early Norse explorers were tempted not by islands that did not exist, but by images of real islands on the horizon to the west!

Outside of polar regions, variations from standard refraction values seldom approach 2 to 3 minutes, occasionally more. In polar regions, refraction variations of a couple of minutes are commonplace and on occasion extreme values of 5 degrees have been reported, which would produce an error of over 300 miles (484 kilometers) in a line of position. It is less than 250 miles (403 kilometers) from the Faroe Islands to Iceland and only another 180 miles (290 kilometers) to Greenland. Could it be that intermittently over the years these islands loomed above the horizon tempting the Norse explorers with "real" mirages? Just possibly this unfair natural advantage explains why the Nordic explorers beat their southern nautical colleagues to the New World by 500 years!

SAILING ACUITY

Although nature has produced a prodigious number of different eyes to meet the needs of its species, there have been two major lines of development. One line has produced a system of *high visual acuity*, which allows the animal to analyze fine visual detail. The culmination of this line of development occurs in the predatory birds, some of whom seem to possess better visual acuity than man. The only drawback to this system is that it requires a lot of light to function, so animals that depend on it to make their living are restricted, for the most part, to a daytime existence.

The other major line has produced a system that sacrifices visual acuity for *visual sensitivity*. This type of eye is designed primarily for a nocturnal existence. It makes maximal use of the meager amount of light available at night. The trade-off is that high visual sensitivity precludes high visual acuity. But a sailor searching for a buoy light or a freighter's running lights, or an animal searching for its predator, is not as interested in fine visual detail as in early apprehension.

The human visual system has borrowed from each of these systems. It is wrong, however, to consider the human eye as a compromise between these extremes. As a compromise, after all, our vision would be best during periods of twilight. Rather, we have incorporated elements of both systems so that in a sense we have four eyes and not two!

Each system has its own specialized receptor. *Cones,* on the one hand, are light-sensitive receptors concentrated in the center of the retina and are responsible for high visual acuity and color vision. *Rods,* on the other hand, are located primarily in the peripheral portions of the retina and are responsible for visual sensitivity (especially at night) and for motion detection. Since most of our sailing life is spent in the daytime when there is adequate illumination, let us first examine our daytime visual system.

Visual acuity is a measure of the ability of the eye to distinguish visual detail, stated in terms of *visual angle.* The visual angle is the angle that light rays coming from the outer limits of an object form at the eye. Figure 8.11*A* illustrates the visual angle that a distant sailboat creates in the retina of the eye. It is small and inverted. Figure 8.11*B* represents either a larger sailboat or the same boat nearer the observer. Thus the size of the visual angle depends upon the size of the object and its distance from the observer.

Figure 8.11*C* illustrates the most common means of quantifying visual

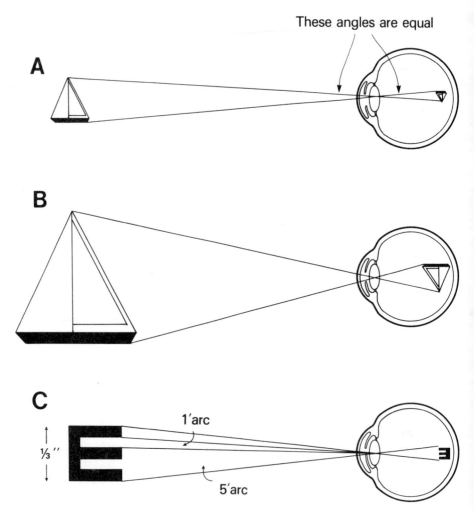

Figure 8.11. *Visual acuity.*

acuity, the eye chart. In the figure, the *E* is one-third of an inch (0.85 centimeter) high, and at a distance of 20 feet (6 meters), the outer limits of the *E* extend under a visual angle of 5 minutes of arc. However, in order to recognize it as an *E*, the detail of the letter (the black bars and white gaps) must be appreciated. Since the bars and gaps represent one-fifth of the overall size of the letter, the minimum detail needed to recognize the letter subtends 1 minute of arc. This detection of detail is called *resolution,* and the eye is said to have a *resolving power* of 1 minute of arc.[11]

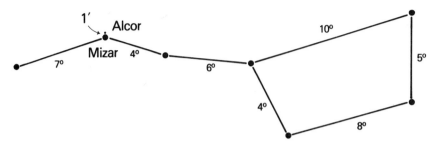

Figure 8.12. Celestial acuity—Alcor and Mizar.

It may surprise you to learn that a similar concept of visual acuity was appreciated in antiquity! Although the ancients did not have an eye chart (the Dutch ophthalmologist Snellen invented it in 1862), they took advantage of what was readily available—the sky. Figure 8.12 illustrates the stars of the Big Dipper, with the distances between the stars rendered in terms of visual angle, equivalent to the angle of a great circle on the celestial sphere. Very close to Mizar, the middle star in the handle, sits a faint, tiny star named Alcor. The distance between these two stars is 1 minute of arc. In the ancient world, resolution of these two stars was equivalent to normal vision. This became part of the Roman "physical" for soldiers. If only one star was seen, vision was subnormal. It is not known whether ancients used other naturally occurring visual parameters to quantify lesser visual acuities.

It might appear at first glance that 1 minute of arc is the best that the eye is capable of, but this is not so. *In fact, for most of us, 20/20 visual acuity is not normal at all.* If tested carefully, most of us are capable of resolving less than 1 minute of arc. We can read the 20/15 or even the 20/13 lines on the eye chart.

For the moment, let us consider 1 minute of arc as a benchmark against which to compare our visual abilities in various nautical situations. In certain circumstances we don't do quite that well, whereas in others we do a bit better.

As a mariner approaches a prominent landmark or buoy from a distance, there are three phases of visual appreciation. The first is when the object is *detected* as distinct from its surroundings (detection range). The object on the horizon is just beyond the resolving power of the eye in minutes of arc. In other words, there is something that could be a buoy—or it might turn out to be a fishing boat! Upon closer approach, it can be *recognized* as an aid to navigation, possessing a certain shape and color (recognition range). At the recognition range, the eye can resolve the dark buoy—analogous to the bar of the *E*—against the lighter gaps of the sky. There is enough information in minutes of arc to indicate that the object is indeed a buoy. Later in the recognition phase, the color of the buoy becomes apparent. Finally, the buoy can be *identified* when the mariner is close enough to read the numbers or letters (identification range). All three ranges—detection, recognition, and identification—depend on the resolving power of the eye, and each presents a different amount of information to the sailor.

BINOCULARS AND OTHER NAUTICAL INSTRUMENTS

When visual discrimination is limited due to the eye's inability to resolve fine detail, binoculars are of value. Binoculars are able to do only one thing—they increase the apparent visual angle of the object and hence the size of the image on the retina. This increases the range of an object such as a buoy by a factor equal to the magnifying power of the binoculars (7 times with 7 x 35 or 7 x 50 binoculars). For example, a buoy that is barely detected may now be recognized with binoculars. The size of the image on the retina is now large enough (usually about 1 minute of arc) for the eye to resolve. Likewise, a buoy within the recognition range may now be identified. It is important to realize that in each of these cases, the contrast between the object and the background is sufficient. Merely the size of the object limits visual resolution. Binoculars are of little or no assistance in situations where the contrast is low, such as in penetrating, dense haze or fog.

Binoculars are not capable of increasing the contrast between the object and its background (in this case the buoy and the horizon). In fact, because all optical instruments introduce a slight amount of light scatter from the surfaces of the lenses, they tend to decrease rather than increase contrast. *Therefore, if visibility conditions set the limit for visual resolution, binoculars are of no use.*

Let us return to our benchmark visual resolution of 1 minute of arc. Ultimately, the sensitivity of the cones depends upon precisely how they are stimulated. In the case of the black and white bars of the eye chart, we can resolve slightly less than 1 minute of arc. If two point sources of light are used (such as Alcor and Mizar), the best possible resolution, using refined astronomical equipment, is 36 seconds of arc. This figure is in close agreement with what would be expected based on the size and separation of the most tightly packed cones in the absolute center of the retina.

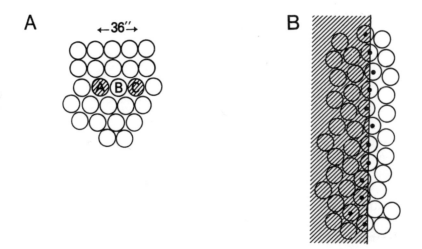

Figure 8.13. Cones in the absolute center of the retina. A. To be recognized as two distinct points of light, the two stimulated cones must be separated by a nonstimulated cone. B. Averaging of cone responses allows vernier acuity, or detection of lines and edges as fine as 3 to 5 seconds of arc.

But if 36 seconds of arc is the best possible resolution, are we deluding ourselves by taking sextant observations at intervals of 0.1 to 0.2 minute (6 to 12 seconds) of arc? Obviously not, and the explanation is that the retinal cones are exquisitely sensitive to lines and edges of objects.

For two points to be resolved, two stimulated cones (A and C, Figure 8.13A) must be separated by a nonstimulated cone (B). The distance between the centers of the two stimulated cones is 36 seconds of arc, which is why 36 seconds represents the limit of two-point resolution. For an edge, however, the distinction between the stimulated and nonstimulated portions can be determined to less than one cone diameter by averaging the responses of all of the cones along the edge (Figure 8.13B). This type of resolution is referred to as *vernier acuity*. It allows detection of lines and edges as fine as 3 to 5 seconds of arc.

The sensitivity to lines and edges explains the precision of the sextant as an optical instrument. Obviously, the precision depends to a large degree on the quality of the instrument; however, with a good sextant, the instrument error should be less than 6 to 12 seconds of arc. Therefore, our sextant observations themselves should approach a vernier acuity, especially with large bright objects such as the sun or moon. It should be approximated by our observations of the stars and planets as well. The unfortunate implication is that we no longer have a valid excuse for poor sextant observations!

COLOR

One question that arose early in the investigation of color was: If the human eye can distinguish among 150 different colors, how many types of cones are there? If each hue were analyzed by a separate cone, the job of packaging 150 different cones would be enormous. If each point on the retina were represented by each of these cones, the "grain" of the color image would be extremely coarse.

Instead, nature subcontracted the work of color discrimination to various portions of the eye and brain. Three types of cones perform the "blue-collar" job of receiving the different wavelengths of light; each type receives a different portion of the light spectrum. The red cone is maximally sensitive to wavelengths around 570 nanometers, the green cone to wavelengths at 535 nanometers, and the blue cone to the shorter wavelengths, which center around 445 nanometers (Figure 8.14). Note that there is a great deal of overlap in the territory that each of the cones serves, so any single wavelength usually stimulates two and sometimes three types of cones. The amount of stimulation of each of the cones determines the color. Other cells in the retina perform the "white-collar" job of sorting out all of this, whereas the "executive-level" decisions regarding color are reserved for the brain.

All of the other hues are produced from the stimulation of two or three cones in different proportions. Mixtures of blue and green wavelengths produce various shades of blue-green, whereas green and red wavelengths produce yellow and orange. Violet results from mixing wavelengths from both ends of the spectrum—blue and red. Note that these rules of color mixing hold only when the colors are *additive,* as are pure spectral bands of light, e.g., the kind of light navigational lights produce at night. If you could superimpose a red and a green navigational light, the resulting light would appear yellow. In a sense, the appearance of the sun during the day is due to such a superimposition since it is missing the scattered blue.[12]

If the eye has a range of approximately 300 nanometers (400 to 700 nanometers) and if within that range more than 150 colors can be distinguished, it follows that the eye must be exquisitely sensitive to very small differences in wavelength. Figure 8.15 demonstrates that the eye is

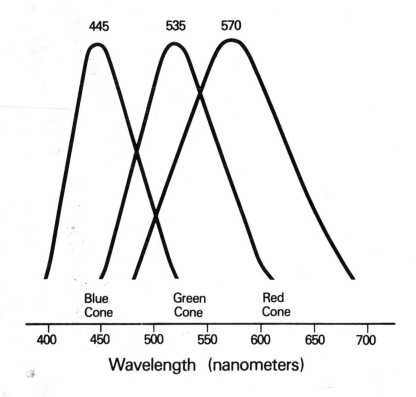

Figure 8.14. The three types of cones: red, green, and blue.

not equally sensitive to all portions of the spectrum. Roughly speaking, it is most sensitive to the portions of the spectrum between the three cone curves, i.e., in the blue-green zone and in the yellow zone, between green and red. In these regions the eye is capable of discriminating colors at 1- nanometer increments! This sensitivity to minute color variations allows us to use changes in the color of the water as natural aids to navigation when sailing in certain regions—often referred to as eyeball navigation. *The Yachtsman's Guide to the Greater Antilles* provides an example of this kind of visual piloting:

> It is almost impossible to describe in words what only experience can really teach, but let us take a stab at it. All of what we say here is assuming there is good light—high and behind the observer—and relatively calm water.
> In depths of over 60 feet the water has a deep "inky" blue-black color. Over sand this color takes on a lighter but still deep blue color—if the bot-

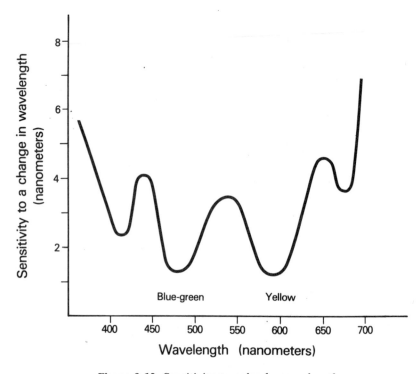

Figure 8.15. *Sensitivity to color by wavelength.*

tom is rocky the color is more of a dark green. On coming into water of about 25 to 30 feet a sandy bottom will show as a light green—if it is a rocky bottom it will be more of a mottled brown color. In going into shallower water the sandy bottom reflects a very pale green at about 10 feet. Over rock or coral at this depth, the water will take on a yellow-brown, mottled tinge and you should be able to distinguish very clearly the outlines of the rocks.[13]

Eyeball navigation is actually superior to traditional depth sounding in several respects. Not only is the eye capable of sampling data over a much greater area, but the sailor can also judge the depth and composition of the bottom before it is—ugh!—beneath his keel. Anyone who wishes to practice eyeball navigation should keep the following points in mind. A good pair of polarized lenses is essential, preferably neutral gray. A hat or visor contributes to diminishing the glare. The visibility is usually good over coral bottoms except after heavy rain when the water may be muddy. Human activities such as dumping, dredging, or blasting may also impair clarity. *Anticipating the time of passage through the reef is absolutely crucial*. Plan to cross the reef only when the sun is high and behind, shining over your shoulder.[14] This means that in the morning you can expect good visibility through water in a westerly direction and in the afternoon in an easterly direction. The higher the sun gets, the wider the "arc" of visibility; the lower the sun, the narrower the arc. Also, if the sun's noontime passage lies to the north of your position, visibility will be somewhat better to the south, and vice versa. If the water is calm and "glassy," it may be difficult to see below the surface. Fortunately, it is rare for the water to be perfectly calm, and even the slightest ripple on the surface enhances vision. Finally, beware of cloud shadows that may resemble coral heads.

There is one other role of color with which the sailor should be familiar—the appreciation of distance. During normal atmospheric conditions, all distant objects such as hills or mountains are lightly veiled in a blue haze due to the preferential scattering of blue light. Through experience we have come to associate this indistinct blue quality with distance (as did Leonardo da Vinci, who first emphasized it as an important technique to create depth perception in painting). When the atmosphere is unusually dry and clear, however, the blue haze is absent and distant objects stand out starkly against the horizon. This starkness creates the illusion of nearness, so distant objects may be interpreted as being much closer than they really are.

TWILIGHT

During twilight the eye is in the embarrassing position of being "between systems."[15] It is still too bright for the nighttime rod system and too dark for the optimal performance of the daytime cone system. Nevertheless, it is an important period for the mariner. It may be the only time of day when the navigator has the opportunity to obtain a fix from simultaneous celestial observations. In addition, if the boat overstands the estimated time of travel, twilight can be an anxious transition period during which everyone worries whether there will be enough light to identify various aids to navigation.

Both the navigator and the helmsman should be aware that the rate of change in illumination is not constant. The brightness of twilight changes relatively slowly until the sun is about 4 degrees below the horizon. From that point on, the decrease in illumination proceeds at an accelerated pace, and visual piloting rapidly becomes a losing battle. Both of the major cone functions needed for piloting—visual acuity and color vision—degrade

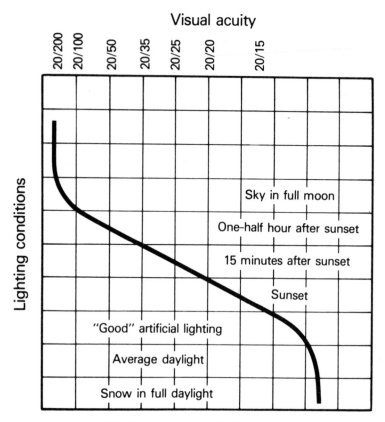

Figure 8.16. The loss of acuity with diminished illumination.

together so that the nautical environment becomes increasingly indistinct and gray. Figure 8.16 illustrates the relationship between visual acuity and illumination. Note that at about a half hour after sunset, visual acuity is reduced to about 20/100, a visual angle of 5 minutes. This means that a daymark that was previously identified at 0.1 nautical mile (185 meters) now has an identification range of 0.03 mile or 190 feet (57 meters).

NIGHTTIME SAILING

The versatility of the eye is truly astonishing if we consider that it is capable of responding to light as dim as 10^{-8} footcandles and as bright as 10^7 footcandles. This remarkable adaptability represents a range of 10^{15} (1,000,000,000,000,000) log units of intensity!

The cone system, which has a higher threshold (i.e., is less sensitive),

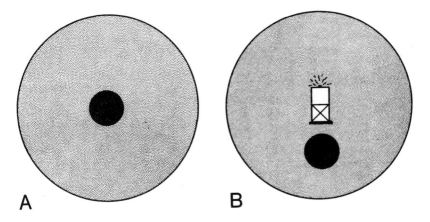

Figure 8.17. The "blind spot."

functions between 10^{-2} footcandles (medium moonlight) and 10^7 foot-candles (intolerably bright light). The rod system, which operates between 10^{-8} and 10^{-2} footcandles, provides the eye with nighttime sensitivity.[16] In exchange we surrender both high visual acuity and all perception of color. With rod vision, the world appears in various shades of black and white. Since there are no rods in the exact center of the retina, in conditions of dim illumination there is a blind spot of about 5 degrees in the center of our visual field (Figure 8.17). No matter where we move our eyes, this blind spot remains. Because of this, *navigators and pilots are trained to look about 5 degrees to one side of (or above or below) the object for which they are searching in the dark.*

The changeover from one system to the other does not occur instantaneously. For example, when passing from the bright sunlight into a darkened movie theater, it is difficult at first to see anything at all. But, after a few minutes, we can see the surroundings fairly well; we have adapted to the dark (dark adaptation). Conversely, on leaving the theater, we are initially dazzled by the bright sunlight and must readapt to the light (light adaptation). Light adaptation is rarely a problem—it occurs in seconds. Dark adaptation, however, requires a longer period of time.

The rod system requires more than 30 minutes to dark-adapt—up to an hour for complete adaptation—but during this time it increases sensitivity by 1 million times! Unfortunately, a few *seconds* of exposure to bright light can undo an entire hour of dark adaptation. For this reason, anyone who wishes to remain dark-adapted must avoid all white light, even cabin light. *Whenever there is a change of watch at night, the reliev-*

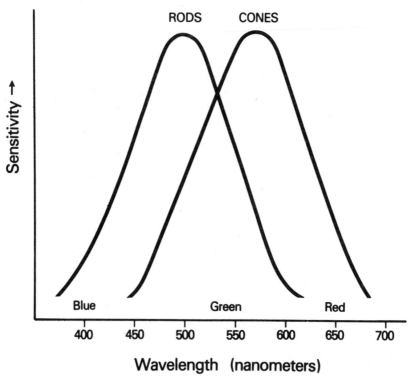

RODS   **CONES**

Sensitivity →

Blue   Green   Red

400   450   500   550   600   650   700

Wavelength (nanometers)

Figure 8.18. Sensitivity of the rods and cones by wavelength.

ing watch should allow 30 minutes to become fully dark-adapted prior to assuming duty.

There is a way to use the high visual acuity system and still retain the rods in a dark-adapted, high-readiness state. This requires the use of monochromatic red light. The rods are insensitive to the long, red wavelengths of light. Figure 8.18 represents the sensitivity curves for both rods and cones. Notice that the curve for the rods is shifted to the left so that most of the red wavelengths are beyond its capabilities. Since there are only 3 types of cones in the center of the retina (instead of, say, 150), they are packed close enough so that it is possible to see just about 20/20 with pure red light without affecting the rods at all.

For this reason, the compass light is red and the prepared mariner has a flashlight with a red filter. In the eventuality that a brief chart consultation is required, the mariner is able to resume duty immediately. An alternative is to use red goggles that filter the light at the eye instead of at the source. Without red light or goggles, another little-known trick may be used, which supports the fact that we really do have four eyes and not two! Dark adaptation is entirely a property of the retina, and each eye dark-adapts independently. Thus, if the navigator is fully dark-adapted and must go below to consult a chart, he can simply close one eye. The covered eye remains dark-adapted. When he returns on deck, he can switch eyes or leave both eyes open. (This trick is also useful when a midnight trip to the head is necessary either on land or at sea.)

One concept needs to be explored further: the relationship between the two systems. It is wrong to visualize the cone system at work only by day and the rod system on a lonely watch at night. During the daytime the cone system is dominant, but the rods are not entirely quiescent. They function primarily as movement detectors in the peripheral visual field. At night the rod system is dominant, but the cone system is poised for action, awaiting an appropriately intense stimulus. Even in starlight the cone system *must* be working; otherwise, we could never distinguish Alcor from Mizar nor could we appreciate the blueness of Venus or the redness of Mars, both properties of the cone system. The key is that the stimulus must be sufficiently intense. Individual stars do not provide much background illumination, but since they are point sources of light, they *intensely* stimulate a small area of the retina, often one or two cones.

In order to appreciate the relationship between these two systems, imagine that you are searching on a clear night for a flashing, green light with a *nominal range* (the maximal distance at which a light can be seen at night when the visibility is clear) of 3 miles (4.9 kilometers). At some distance beyond the nominal range, perhaps at 4 miles (6.4 kilometers), the rod system may detect the light. At this stage the approximate direction of the light is apparent, but a precise bearing is not possible. All the same, this information may prove useful. At perhaps 3.5 miles (5.6 kilometers), the light will be intense enough to stimulate the cones (allowing a bearing), *but the light will appear white.* The period after a light is visible as white but before its color is appreciated is known as the *photochromatic interval.* It is characteristic of all colored lights at night. At the nominal range of the light, in this case 3 miles (4.9 kilometers), all of its characteristics including color will be apparent.

The scenario is similar for a red light, with one exception. If the lights were of the same intensity, the red light would be invisible at 4 miles (6.4 kilometers) because the rod system is insensitive to red light. At about 3.5 miles (5.6 kilometers), it would be visible to the cone system as a white light, and after the photochromatic interval it would appear red.

In many respects, finding a navigational light at night is an easier proposition than finding that same aid to navigation by day since there are fewer variables. By day, the variables include the size, shape, color, and reflectivity of the object; the background against which it is seen; the elevation and angular relationship of the sun and object; the general level of illumination, including cloud cover and glare; visibility conditions; and the height of the observer's eye.

At night there are only three variables: the power of the *light,* the *visibility*, and the *position of the observer's eye* relative to the light. If it were not for one of these variables, we could see any light in the hemisphere at any time!

It is axiomatic that a powerful light will be seen at a greater distance than will a weak one, but why? The explanation is that even during conditions of normal visibility, the atmosphere impedes the progress of light waves. After all, the only reason we are able to see the stars is that they spend 99.999... percent of their journey traveling through interstellar space, which is so rarefied that there are few molecules with which the light can collide. This is certainly not the case on earth. Therefore, one limiting factor or variable is the strength of the light, or its nominal range.

If the visibility is normal, only one factor can prevent the light from reaching the observer: the relationship between the height of the light and the height of the observer's eye. This relationship, known as the *geographic range,* is purely geometric and has nothing to do with the power of the light. Since the earth is curved and since light *usually* travels in a straight line, there is a distance beyond which the light is below the horizon of the observer. Bowditch provides this information in tabulated form.[17] The formula for calculating distance to the horizon (for both eye and light) is

$$D = 1.144\sqrt{h},$$

where D is the distance in nautical miles and h is the height of either the light or the observer's eye. *On a clear night one of these two factors determines when a light is visible to the sailor.*

What if the visibility is reduced? Lowered visibility has no effect on the geographic range, but it does have an impact on the strength of the light since the "thicker" the atmosphere, the more difficult it is for the light rays to penetrate. The strength of the light, corrected for prevailing visibility conditions, is known as the *luminous range* and can be determined from a luminous range diagram such as the one provided in any volume of the United States Light List.

With this in mind, estimating the expected appearance of a light at night becomes downright straightforward. In clear visibility the limiting factor will be either (1) the power of the light (nominal range) or (2) the geographic range. With reduced visibility the limiting factor will be either (1) the reduced power of the light (luminous range) or (2) the geographic range.

NOTES

1. As sailors we utilize a substantial portion of the electromagnetic spectrum for a variety of purposes (Figure 4.1). The velocity of all electromagnetic radiation is the same, 3 x 10⁸ meters per second (186,000 miles per second). The only difference between, say, light, ultraviolet radiation, and radio waves is their wavelength. The omega navigational system, for example, employs electromagnetic radiation of extremely long wavelength—approximately 10,000 meters long. Radio beacons, Loran, and VHF radio equipment produce energy of progressively shorter wavelength. Each of these systems is designed to transmit or receive energy only in a limited band. To a VHF radio, medium-frequency and high-frequency radiation simply does not exist. So it is with the human eye. It is sensitive to a mere octave in the grand electromagnetic scale. Looked at in this fashion, we are nearly blind.

2. If light is reflected, the angle of the reflected ray is equal to the angle of the incident ray such that angle i (incident ray) equals angle r (reflected ray). It should be kept in mind that with both reflection and refraction, all angles are measured from the perpendicular (normal) to the surface and not from the surface up. The degree of refraction depends on the angle of incidence as well as the index of refraction of the two media, in this case air (1.000) and water (1.333). (This is known as Snell's law, the mathematical expression of which is $n \sin I = n' \sin I'$, where n and n' are the indices of refraction of the two media and $\sin I$ and $\sin I'$ are the sines of the angles of incidence and refraction, respectively.)

3. The primary colors of wavelengths of light are blue, green, and red. Yellow is composed of a mixture of green and red light. If this seems odd, that is because many of us have been raised to conceptualize color only in terms of pigment mixture, a somewhat different system. Color is discussed more fully later in the chapter.

4. *The Nautical Almanac* (Washington: U.S. Government Printing Office; London: Her Majesty's Stationery Office, 1981).

5. A. B. Fraser and W. H. Mach, "Mirages," *Scientific American* 234 (1976):102-111.

6. Ibid.

7. Sir Francis Chichester, *Gipsy Moth Circles the World* (Sevenoaks: Hodder and Stoughton, and New York: Coward-McCann, l967), p. 206.

8. Fraser and Mach, "Mirages."

9. S. E. Morison, *The European Discovery of America: The Northern Voyages,* p. 103.

10. Ibid., p. 101.

11. The visual acuity fraction we commonly use is simply a numerical expression of the resolving power of the eye:

$$\text{Visual acuity} = \frac{\text{Distance at which the test is made (usually 20 feet)}}{\text{Distance at which the minimum detail of the smallest recognized letter is 1 minute of arc}}$$

The detail in the E in Figure 8.11C subtends 1 minute of arc at 20 feet and, if recognized, visual acuity is 20/20. The big E at the top of most eye charts has visual detail that subtends 1 minute of arc at 200 feet, and if it is the smallest letter that can be recognized, then visual acuity is 20/200, very poor indeed.

12. By comparison, a paint gains color because its pigment absorbs all of the

wavelengths of light *except* those that are reflected. A red buoy appears red because the paint absorbs the blue and green wavelengths while reflecting the red wavelengths to the eye. The mixing of pigments is referred to as *subtractive* color mixing. The empiric rules of mixing are different in the two cases, but the principles are the same if one considers only the light that reaches the eye.

13. H. Kline, ed., *Yachtsman's Guide to the Greater Antilles* (Coral Gables: Tropic Isle, 1979), pp. 135-136.

14. With the sun behind you, there is significantly less glare with which to contend. Unless the sun is relatively high, there are too few light rays reflected off the coral toward the observer, and those that are reflected stand a good chance of undergoing total internal reflection (see Figure 8.5).

15. Twilight is so important that various groups have defined it according to their own interests and needs; thus we have three different twilight periods: civil, nautical, and astronomic. The duration of *civil twilight,* a time in which there is still sufficient light for most terrestrial outdoor activities, is defined as that interval between the time when the upper edge of the sun is on, and the true position of its center is 6 degrees below, the horizon. *Nautical twilight* is longer, since there is a longer period of light at sea than on land due to the lack of obstructions such as mountains and the reflectivity of the water. Nautical twilight lasts from sunset until the sun is 12 degrees below the horizon. *Astronomic twilight* is still longer, since astronomers are interested in knowing when the sky will be dark enough for star observation. The darker limit of astronomic twilight occurs when the sun is 18 degrees beneath the horizon.

16. When nature set about to build a high-sensitivity system, she not only succeeded, but in the end created *the most sensitive system possible.* In order to appreciate the sensitivity of the rod system, we must ultimately reexamine the nature of light itself and redress an egregious error of omission. Earlier, light was considered exclusively as a wave phenomenon. But to stop there belies the dual nature of light and glosses over one of the classic controversies in the history of science. For over 300 years, there were two rival theories of the nature of light. On one side was the imposing figure of Isaac Newton (1642-1727), who argued that light must be composed of a train of particles. His adversary and contemporary was Christian Huygens (1629-1695), who maintained that light behaved primarily as a series of waves. The battle raged on, and for a time it looked as though Newton's theory of particles was wrong. However, at the beginning of the 20th century it was shown conclusively that the wave theory could not explain all of the characteristics of light. It is now clear that light is both particle *and* wave. Sometimes the behavior of light is best described by its wave motions, while under other conditions it is best considered to be composed of particles or *photons.* A photon is the smallest possible parceling of light energy. Amazingly, the rod is capable of responding, under ideal conditions, to a single photon of light! The system is so sensitive that it can be stimulated by the smallest quantity of light possible in our universe. To be fair, a single photon doesn't produce a visual sensation. This requires the activation of at least two, perhaps as many as five, rods at the same time.

17. N. Bowditch, *American Practical Navigator* (Washington: Defense Mapping Agency Hydrographic Center, 1975), vol. 2, p. 132.

9

Keeping in Shape

*Seafaring people are that class of
mankind who are supposed to be in perfect
health when they enroll themselves for any
particular voyage or cruise; notwithstand-
ing their hardiness, they are liable to
many and numerous excruciating maladies....
Sailors are very apt to become careless
of their health, especially while in port,
and expose themselves to every intemper-
ance that can possibly produce the
occasional causes of disease.*

Samuel H. P. Lee, M.D. and Apothecary, 1795

EVERY SAILOR HAS A reason to keep in shape. The small-boat-racing sailor recognizes that sailing is like any other sport that requires a high degree of training and physical conditioning. He is interested in developing an exercise program that improves flexibility while strengthening those muscle groups crucial to the small-boat racer—primarily the muscles of the back and torso. Crew members of larger boats, by contrast, may wish to design an exercise program that focuses on upper-body strength. Grinding or tailing a winch requires short, repetitive bursts of power. Their exercises differ in many fundamental respects from those of the small-boat racer. The cruising sailor may not have any interest in training for competition. Nevertheless, there are other reasons for keep-

---

TABLE 9.1
Risk Factors

Primary-Risk Factors
- High Blood Pressure
- Hyperlipidemia
  (High Fat and/or Cholesterol)
- Cigarette Smoking

Secondary-Risk Factors
- Family History of Cardiovascular Disease
  (Heart Attack, Stroke)
- Prolonged Physical Inactivity
- Obesity
- Diabetes Mellitus

---

ing in shape. For one thing, exercise improves the overall efficiency of the human machinery, making it less vulnerable to injury or accident. Additionally, most people simply feel better when they are engaged in a regular exercise program.

It is important for the mariner to tailor an exercise program that reflects both his specific goals as well as his individual constraints of time and space. An exercise program, after all, is time-consuming, and most of us have to choose from a myriad of exercises those that will further clearly identified goals. Exercises chosen willy-nilly take time with little demonstrable effect. Space may also be a consideration. Many of the exercises discussed here require heavy equipment. Since there is no place for such equipment aboard a sailboat, the cruising sailor is forced to plan ahead and seek imaginative alternatives. When designing a program, the sailor should identify specific goals: *strength, flexibility, speed,* or *endurance.* Individual programs emphasize one or more of these goals. The importance of identifying in advance those goals that are primary and those that are secondary cannot be overemphasized.

What precautions should be taken prior to commencing an exercise program? If the sailor is less than 35 years of age, has no history of cardiovascular disease, and has no known primary-risk factors (see Table 9.1), he can begin without formal medical clearance (although many physicians still advise an evaluation within the previous 2 years). Secondary-risk factors by themselves do not imply the need for further pre-exercise evaluation. If the sailor is younger than 35 but has a significant combination of risk factors, it is best to obtain medical clearance including an exercise-stress electrocardiogram. Everyone over the age of 35 who is either beginning an exercise program or increasing his exercise habits to an appreciable extent should be so tested.

TRAINING THEORY

There are four basic exercise concepts that the sailor should consider when designing his individualized exercise program.

The program must incorporate a specific exercise overload in order to bring about improvement. The *overload principle* applies to both aerobic and anaerobic exercises. In order to improve biceps strength using arm curls, for example, there must be enough weight to overload the biceps (see Figure 9.12). Multiple repetitions with a light weight that doesn't overload the biceps results in little or no improvement. Similarly, aerobic exercises such as running or swimming must be performed at a level significantly above normal to produce a positive, lasting effect on the cardiorespiratory system. The degree of overload for any exercise can be varied by manipulating its *intensity, frequency,* or *duration.*

Individuality is also a factor in the training program. Clearly, if exercise must overload the system, the absolute exercise level varies from individual to individual according to his or her relative fitness at the start of the training. The amount of aerobic exercise needed to overload the cardiorespiratory system is markedly different for a marathon runner, a sedentary adult, and a cardiac patient! *The benefits of any training program are optimized when the program is planned to meet individual needs and capabilities.*

The *specificity principle* is the least understood of the training concepts. This is unfortunate, since misunderstanding of this concept has resulted in much wasted time and unrealistic expectations. Simply stated, *specific exercises produce specific changes in the body that result in specific improvements in performance.* Since the improvements in performance are specific for the type of exercise performed, the sailor should try to formulate an exercise program that mimics the kinds of activities he will need to perform. Many sailors want to concentrate on anaerobic activities that improve strength. Aerobic activities such as running, swimming, or bicycling may add little or nothing to the sailor's performance.[1] It is a fallacy that aerobic training makes the sailor "more fit" or "in better shape" to perform any and all activities. Unless the task the sailor must carry out has an aerobic component, being aerobically fit will not improve his performance one bit. Although most sailing tasks are primarily or exclusively anaerobic, some of the highly competitive racing sailors probably can benefit from aerobic training. In addition, the sailor may have some other reason to perform aerobic exercises.

The fourth principle is the *reversibility principle.* After only 2 weeks of "detraining," significant reductions in exercise performance are observed. Almost all of the training improvement is lost within several months. Thus, the beneficial effects of exercise are both transient and reversible. For this reason, the program must be *realistic.* Only then is there a possibility that it will be incorporated into the weekly schedule.[2]

TRAINING FOR STRENGTH

Most of the popular forms of strength training are variations on a program of *progressive resistance exercises,* or PRE. PRE exercises consist of three variables: the amount of weight that can be lifted (measured in pounds of resistance), the number of repetitions (usually 8 to 15), and the number of sets of repetitions (usually three).

The first step in performing PRE is to determine (or estimate), for each exercise, the maximum amount of weight that can be lifted on a one-time basis. This maximum weight is not employed in training since excessive weight contributes little to the development of strength and greatly increases the likelihood of muscle and joint injury. Rather, 70 to 75 percent of the maximum should be used. If the maximum weight that can be lifted in a bench press, for example, is 100 pounds (45 kilograms), only 70 to 75 pounds (32 to 34 kilograms) should be used initially for that exercise. This weight is still too heavy if the exerciser cannot perform 12 repetitions. However, if the repetitions feel too easy, a heavier weight should be selected. Determining the initial weight is a process of trial and error. The goal is to complete three sets of 12 repetitions. After 1 to 2 weeks of training, when the muscles have adapted and the correct movements are second nature, the target number of repetitions can be decreased to 8 to 10. The weight will then have to be adjusted periodically as the muscles become stronger. Increments of 5 pounds (2.25 kilograms) for the arms and 10 pounds (4.5 kilograms) for the legs are suggested. The PRE program can be performed with individual weights (see figures in this chapter) or on a machine such as the Universal.

PRE is a form of *isotonic* strength training. Isotonic contraction involves either a shortening or a lengthening of the muscle against a fixed resistance. Two other forms of strength training are available: isometric and isokinetic exercise.

Isometric strength training differs from isotonics in that the length of the muscle and the angle of the joint do not change when contraction takes place. If the sailor attempts to push or lift an object that he cannot move, his muscles would be in a state of isometric contraction. In general, isometric exercises are not that valuable. First, they are time-consuming. A contraction must be held at each and every angle of the joint through its entire range, because the strength developed is specific to the joint angle at which contraction takes place. In addition, isometrics is not effective for developing speed of contraction. The *kind* of strength that is developed with isometrics is best suited for isometric tasks (the specificity principle). They are not, for the most part, the kinds of tasks the sailor must perform.

Isokinetic strength training (also known as accommodating resistance exercises, or ARE) has become familiar through the Nautilus isokinetic program. With this method, the machine varies the resistance throughout the entire range of the exercise; that is, every effort encounters an equal and opposing force. This is not true of isotonics, where the greatest force is generated in the initial part of the movement when inertia is overcome. Fewer repetitions are needed with isokinetics—three sets of five to six repetitions would be adequate for each exercise.

Which is superior, isotonics or isokinetics? The question is useful only if we add, For what purpose? For weight-lifting tasks, isotonics is superior to isokinetics since it more nearly imitates the task (the specificity principle, again). However, most of the sailor's tasks (such as grinding a winch, tailing, sweating a halyard, or weighing an anchor) produce continuous resistance throughout the entire range of motion. Isokinetics more closely imitates this kind of resistance, suggesting that isokinetics *may* be superior to isotonics for most boat-related tasks. The advantage, however, is probably slight, and if isotonics is more readily available, the sailor should not despair!

Which specific strength exercises are the most appropriate? This depends on the task or tasks that must be performed. Grinding a winch requires rapid, repetitive bursts of upper-body strength against increasing amounts of resistance. Strong lower back and leg muscles are also needed. Figures 9.12 to 9.18 illustrate a number of exercises designed to strengthen the upper body. They can be performed with standard weights or with isotonic or isokinetic equipment. Instead of the shoulder exercise in Figure 9.18, the sailor can substitute an arm-bicycling program. Simply invert a bicycle and pedal with the arms. The degree of resistance can be adjusted by altering the brake calipers. Approximately 5 minutes probably constitutes

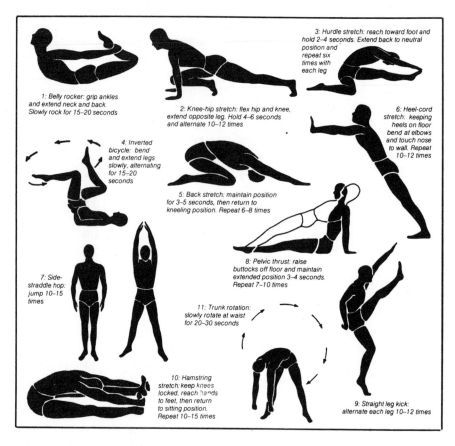

Figures 9.1-9.11. *Warm-up and cool-down exercises. These are calisthenics and stretching exercises and should be done before and after performing any aerobic or progressive resistance exercises. Reproduced, by permission, from Carl E. Klafs and D. Arnheim,* Modern Principles of Athletic Training, *3rd and 4th eds. (St. Louis: C. V. Mosby, 1973, 1974).*

a productive session. Again, the specificity principle suggests that the more closely an exercise mimics the task, the better the ultimate performance.

Winch tailers may wish to use some of the exercises for grinders, but they should concentrate on those illustrated in Figures 9.19 to 9.21. In addition, they should consider wrist- and hand-strengthening exercises such as supination-pronation (palm up—palm down) exercises with dumbbells, wrist rolling (down-and-back) exercises, and any other exercise that strengthens handgrip. Repetitive squeezing of a rubber ball is excellent

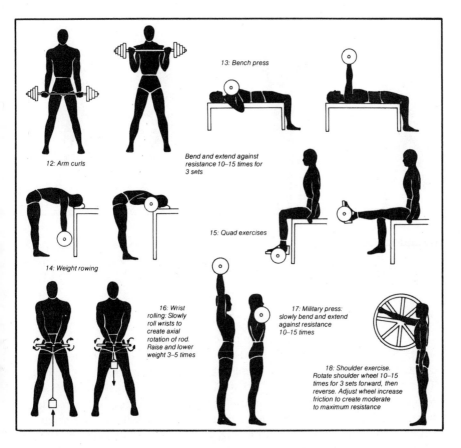

Figures 9.12-9.18. Progressive resistance exercises that can be used by winch grinders. Reproduced, by permission, from Carl E. Klafs and D. Arnheim, Modern Principles of Athletic Training, *4th ed. (St. Louis: C. V. Mosby, 1974).*

and can be accomplished anywhere. Rope or pole climbing is also worth adding to the routine.

Small-boat sailors who must hike out or use a trapeze require special exercises to strengthen the lower back, abdomen, and legs (Figures 9.22 to 9.26). Those sailors who have experienced backache in the past may wish to preface this program with a sequence of basic low-back exercises (see Figure 9.27 and discussion later in this chapter).

In designing a strength-power program, the sailor should incorporate a number of general principles. Strength training should ideally commence

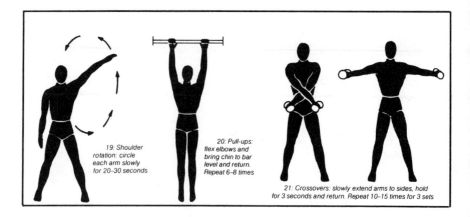

19: Shoulder
rotation: circle
each arm slowly
for 20–30 seconds

20: Pull-ups:
flex elbows and
bring chin to bar
level and return.
Repeat 6–8 times

21: Crossovers: slowly extend arms to sides, hold
for 3 seconds and return. Repeat 10–15 times for 3 sets

Figures 9.19-9.21. *Exercises that can be used by tailers. Additional training should involve rope and/or pole climbing. Reproduced, by permission, from Carl E. Klafs and D. Arnheim,* Modern Principles of Athletic Training, *4th ed. (St. Louis: C. V. Mosby, 1974).*

3 or 4 months before the beginning of the competitive season. Each strength session should be preceded by a 10-to-15-minute *warm-up phase* consisting of calisthenics and stretching exercises (Figures 9.1 to 9.11). The purpose of the warm-up is threefold: it (1) raises the core body temperature, (2) raises deep muscle temperature, and (3) stretches ligaments, tendons, and muscles to permit greater flexibility (see discussion on flexibility training). Following the strength-power session, 10 to 15 minutes should be spent in *cool-down* activity, which may consist of any moderately performed exercise or another session of calisthenics. The cool-down activity allows the cardiorespiratory system to return to its usual level, while preventing the pooling of blood within the muscles (which would otherwise promote muscle stiffness).

If the specificity principle is carried to its logical end, the best training for any sport consists of practicing the event over and over again. Although this is undoubtedly true, many sailors do not have the luxury of continuous on-the-water training! Nevertheless, it is important to replicate the speed, strength, and duration of the tasks that will be performed. Grinding, for example, consists of bursts of effort. Either the shoulder exercise (Figure 9.18) or arm bicycling should be practiced with repetitive brief bursts against a moderate resistance. Since hiking-out requires prolonged muscle contractions, these exercises should be performed more slowly and deliberately.

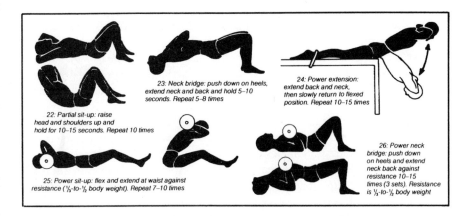

22: Partial sit-up: raise head and shoulders up and hold for 10–15 seconds. Repeat 10 times

23: Neck bridge: push down on heels, extend neck and back and hold 5–10 seconds. Repeat 5–8 times

24: Power extension: extend back and neck, then slowly return to flexed position. Repeat 10–15 times

25: Power sit-up: flex and extend at waist against resistance (⅓-to-½ body weight). Repeat 7–10 times

26: Power neck bridge: push down on heels and extend neck back against resistance 10–15 times (3 sets). Resistance is ⅓-to-½ body weight

Figures 9.22-9.26. Exercises useful for those involved in hiking-out maneuvers. Reproduced, by permission, from Carl E. Klafs and D. Arnheim, Modern Principles of Athletic Training, *4th ed. (St. Louis: C. V. Mosby, 1974).*

How often should strength exercises be performed? The optimum number of training sessions per week is unknown. If a number of different exercises are planned, most authorities suggest two to three sessions per week. There is some evidence that the off days permit healing of the microscopic muscle tears that are inevitable in any vigorous exercise program.

AEROBIC TRAINING

Although weight training produces an improvement in muscle strength, it has no significant influence on the cardiorespiratory system. This is because all of the activities discussed so far are of the anaerobic type. Anaerobic activities—such as winch grinding, swim sprints, and power weight lifts—are typically of short duration, lasting less than 2 minutes. These activities require the immediate release of stored energy sources, such as high-energy compounds adenosine triphosphate (ATP) and creatine phosphate, and the partial breakdown of glucose into the "waste product" lactic acid. If the activity lasts longer than 2 to 4 minutes, aerobic reactions become the major source of energy; and for pure endurance activities like marathon running or distance swimming, they are virtually the sole supplier.

Many sailors consider aerobic training an integral part of their exercise program. Certainly, no one would dispute the fact that aerobic training contributes to their overall level of conditioning, especially the efficiency of their cardiorespiratory system. Nevertheless, we should not lose sight of the fact that *the vast majority of sailing tasks contain little or no aerobic activity.* An exception would be the anaerobic activities of the racing sailor, which must be performed in such rapid succession that they become aerobic.

Aerobic training includes such activities as running, swimming, and bicycling for extended periods of time under conditions that stress the cardiorespiratory system. This level of stress is reached if the exercise is intense enough to increase the heart rate 70 to 85 percent of the individual's *maximum heart rate.* The zone of 70 to 85 percent maximum heart rate is known as the training sensitive zone. Maximum heart rate is conveniently determined by the rule-of-thumb: 220 minus the person's age. Thus, if a 40-year-old man wished to train at moderate intensity above threshold, a training heart rate would be selected that was 70 percent of his maximum predicted heart rate, i.e., 126 beats per minute (220 − 40 = 180 x 0.70 = 126). Then, by trial and error, he would arrive at the running or cycling intensity that produced the desired heart rate. If he wished to train at 85 percent maximum, his exercise heart rate would have to increase to 153 beats per minute (220 − 40 = 180 x 0.85 = 153). Superintense training at heart rates above 85 percent maximum should be discouraged. There are no further gains, whereas there may be "losses." If swimming is chosen for aerobic training—and endurance swimming has potential utility for the sailor—an adjustment is needed in order to estimate maximum heart rate. In swimming, the maximum heart rate is about 13 beats per minute slower than in running, an effect that may be due to the horizontal position of the body and/or the cooling effect of the water. Consequently, that same 40-year-old who wished to swim at 70 percent maximum would select a swimming speed that increased his heart rate to 117 (220 − 40 = 180 − 13 = 167 x 0.70 = 117).

The sailor can determine his heart rate by taking his pulse every 4 to 6 minutes during exercise. The easiest place to take the pulse is over the carotid artery located on either side of the neck. The radial artery on the wrist is another option. Simply count the number of beats in a 10-second period and multiply by 6 (or in a 15-second period and multiply by 4) to obtain the heart rate.

It is advisable to flank the aerobic session with 10-to-15-minute warm-up and cool-down phases. The duration of each aerobic session should be at least 20 to 30 minutes, and 3 to 5 workouts per week are needed to produce cardiorespiratory improvement. Sailors who wish to do both anaerobic and aerobic training may alternate the two.

FLEXIBILITY TRAINING

Improved flexibility is an important part of any conditioning program. Studies have shown that improved flexibility tends to decrease joint injury. It also contributes to improved performance. For the small-boat sailor who must contort his body into a number of unnatural postures, the value of flexibility is obvious. But even the sailor whose main interest is strength training has need for flexibility. Without it, the increase in muscle bulk may diminish the ultimate range of motion, producing "muscle boundness." The concept of muscle boundness is controversial. Whether or not it exists, as a problem it is overrated. Nevertheless, if the sailor engages only in strength-power exercises, the enormous bulk and inelasticity of the muscles, ligaments, and tendons may reduce joint flexibility and mobility.

Two types of exercises improve flexibility: *ballistic* and *static* stretching. In a ballistic stretch, body momentum is utilized to force the muscles into a position of as much stretch as can be tolerated. The hurdler's stretch (Figure 9.3), for example, is often performed with a bobbing of the trunk toward the extended leg in order to stretch the hamstrings. There is evidence that, although this exercise increases flexibility, it induces muscle tears as a consequence of misjudging the stretch tolerance.

Static, or gradual, stretching is now the preferred method. The body is stretched and the position held for a variable period of time, usually 10 to 30 seconds. At the end point, there should be a mild feeling of "tension," but extreme pain must be avoided. The body is relaxed and then stretched again. During the stretching, breathing should be slow, deep, and rhythmic. This helps loosen tight muscles. Most sailors are satisfied with 10-to-15-minute sessions of flexibility exercises during the warm-up and cool-down phases (Figures 9.1 to 9.11). Small-boat-racing sailors may wish to concentrate more heavily in this area.

CIRCUIT TRAINING

Circuit training (CT) is a conditioning technique that combines aspects of both anaerobic and aerobic training. Although there are numerous variations, all CT programs employ a series of 6 to 12 exercise stations arranged in a circuit, often located around the perimeter of an exercise area. Each station is designed for either a calisthenic exercise or a weight-training exercise. The exercises are chosen to address the specific needs of the sailor. The emphasis in CT is on more repetitions (12 to 15) and less weight (40 to 60 percent maximum) than in PRE training. Speed becomes an important factor since the subject moves from one station to another with only a minimal rest of 15 to 30 seconds between stations. The total is one circuit. Two or three circuits is common practice, and the total workout time is generally between 25 and 30 minutes. The lack of rest between stations ensures that the cardiorespiratory system is stressed.

Since CT represents a compromise between pure anaerobic and pure aerobic training, it does not produce as great a gain as when each technique is performed individually. Thus, if the sailor's major concern is to increase strength, he should still consider PRE (see earlier discussion). However, although CT does not produce as much strength as PRE, it contributes to the development of both speed and endurance. Consequently, CT may be attractive to those racing sailors (e.g.,12-meter crews) who must intermittently perform "spurt" activities, such as grinding or tailing, for prolonged periods of time. In this situation, even though each spurt is short, endurance becomes a factor.

What about aerobic improvement with CT? Recent studies have shown that the aerobic intensity during CT is at the minimum threshold level for improving cardiorespiratory fitness. CT should not be considered an adequate aerobic program. However, once the desired stage of fitness is reached through pure aerobic exercise, it can be maintained with less effort through CT. Thus, the racing sailor can build an aerobic base during the off-season and successfully maintain it with CT during the racing season.[3] The cruising sailor who wishes to maintain his aerobic capacity despite being at sea for a prolonged period of time may also consider a CT program.

CRUISING AND CONDITIONING

If motivated, the racing sailor can readily incorporate a shoreside exercise program into his daily routine. The equipment required for strength exercises is often available at a nearby gym or health club, or it can be purchased. Likewise, the only limitation to aerobic conditioning on shore is motivation. On an extended cruise, however, greater limitations are placed on exercise. Unless the sailor prepares, an extended cruise will interfere with his established exercise program, and after a few weeks at sea, he will be in worse shape than when he set sail!

The amount of exercise that the cruising sailor typically receives is deceivingly small. It appears greater than it is because of the muscle soreness and joint stiffness that often accompany an extended cruise. These are due to the limited space on board many cruising boats, which restricts normal, fluid body movements, and to the need to adopt fixed positions for extended periods of time. Furthermore, the distribution of exercise may be unusual. The arms and back typically perform an unaccustomed amount of work, while the legs are underexercised!

What is needed is an individualized, boat-oriented exercise program. The flexibility exercises (Figures 9.1 to 9.11) are easily accomplished. They require no equipment and can be performed, with slight modification, within the confines of even a small boat. Aerobic exercises, at the other extreme, present a formidable challenge. As we have seen, however, aerobics adds little or nothing to the cruising sailor's performance and for that reason can be dispensed with; the sailor can stay healthy and in good shape without aerobics. The real problem arises when the sailor is engaged in aerobics for another reason—perhaps weight control, a second athletic activity, or a desire for improved cardiorespiratory "tone"—and wishes to continue it at sea. If it is a blue-water cruise, there is virtually no opportunity except for jumping rope or running in place. Obviously, distance running, swimming, and bicycling are out unless the passages are short and the sailor can go ashore. By and large, circuit training probably represents the most feasible method to maintain aerobic fitness on a blue-water cruise.

Strength-power training requires compromises and imagination. On larger boats and on ships, it may be practical to bring a set of barbells, but on many boats adjustable dumbbells are an acceptable compromise. Men should bring up to 30 pounds (13.5 kilograms) or more (depending on their initial strength), women somewhat less. Many of the strength exercises can be adapted for dumbbells (Figures 9.12 to 9.14, 9.17, 9.25, and 9.26). Weight rowing (Figure 9.14) is best done with dumbbells by bringing both weights up and out to the side.

Pushups are also worth adding to the upper-body regimen. By varying the distance between the hands, much of the shoulder musculature can be strengthened.

A chin-up bar (Figure 9.20) can be constructed easily from a 30-to-36-inch (75-to-90-centimeter) long, 1-inch (2.5-centimeter) diameter hardwood dowel. A 1/2-inch (1.25-centimeter) line should be secured to both ends, knotted at the midpoint, and fastened to a halyard.

Sit-ups are quite useful for conditioning the back, abdomen, and thigh muscles. Deep knee bends with resistance (barbells or dumbbells) are excellent for strengthening the legs. Exercise aficionados might even consider arm dips on the companionway; the only limit for the cruising sailor is his imagination!

Figure 9.27. *Exercises for low back pain.* (*Courtesy McNeil Pharmaceutical*)

1

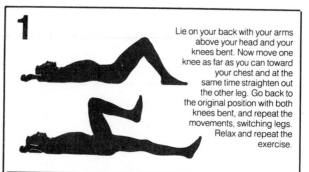

Lie on your back with your arms above your head and your knees bent. Now move one knee as far as you can toward your chest and at the same time straighten out the other leg. Go back to the original position with both knees bent, and repeat the movements, switching legs. Relax and repeat the exercise.

2

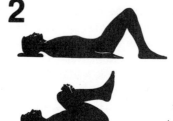

Lie on your back with a small pillow under your head, your arms at your sides and your knees bent. Now bring your knees up to your chest, and with your hands clasped pull your knees toward your chest. Hold for a count of 10, keeping your knees together and your shoulders flat on the mat. Repeat the pulling and holding movement three times. Relax and repeat the exercise.

3

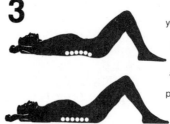

Relax with your arms above your head and your knees bent. Now tighten the muscles of your lower abdomen and your buttocks at the same time so as to flatten your back against the mat. This is the **flat back position**. Hold the position for a count of 10. Relax and repeat the exercise.

4

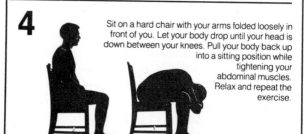

Sit on a hard chair with your arms folded loosely in front of you. Let your body drop until your head is down between your knees. Pull your body back up into a sitting position while tightening your abdominal muscles. Relax and repeat the exercise.

BACKACHE PREVENTION

Backache is probably the most frequent preventable health annoyance among sailors. When sailing, there is an unaccustomed strain on the back muscles during such activities as heavy lifting, stooping, twisting, and just plain sitting in an uncomfortable position for hours at a time. Many sailors, in fact, do not have significant backache anywhere *except* at sea.

Serious causes of backache are usually not the problem—they represent less than 10 percent of the cases. The prime culprit is poor physical conditioning; thus the most vulnerable sailor is the weekend zealot who has not been engaged in regular physical activity. While sedentary, muscle fibers shorten and lose their flexibility. If these shortened, inflexible muscles are suddenly overstretched, the result is predictable—painful muscle tears. These tears produce muscle spasm, which produces more pain, more spasm, and on and on in a vicious cycle.

Engaging in exercises that improve both strength and flexibility can prevent muscle tear and spasm. In fact, many sailors who have been involved in a regular exercise program confirm that the likelihood of backache is inversely related to their degree of physical fitness. When they exercise they do not experience backache. Unfortunately, as soon as the sailor feels better, he is apt to forgo the exercises and return to his sedentary routine, only to be rudely confronted with a recurrence of backache the next time around.

What can be done to avoid this? The sailor who knows that he has a vulnerable back or has just recovered from an attack of backache should begin with exercises specifically designed for low-back disorders (Figure 9.27). It is important not to overdo these exercises, especially in the beginning. Perform the movements slowly and deliberately. There should be very little stiffness after doing these, although there may be *mild* discomfort that lasts a few minutes. If the pain is moderate or severe and lasts more than 15 minutes, discontinue the exercises. It is best to do these exercises on a hard surface covered with a thin mat or heavy blanket. Place a pillow under the head if it is more comfortable. Begin exercises slowly to allow the muscles to loosen up gradually. Plan to work up to 10 repetitions of each.

If you tolerate these exercises well, proceed to leg raises and sit-ups. Leg raises are performed by lying face up and raising both legs a couple of inches off the floor, keeping the knees straight. Hold this position for a few seconds or until it produces discomfort. Gradually increase to 10 repetitions. Sit-ups are next. They should always be done with the knees slightly bent.

Sailors who do a great deal of hiking-out or trapeze work should practice the specific exercises illustrated earlier (Figures 9.22 to 9.26). All of the exercises designed to prevent backache, as well as those for hiking-out, address two main muscle groups: the paraspinal (back and neck) muscles and the abdominal muscles. It is sometimes not appreciated that the abdominal muscles play a major role in preventing backache. With proper hiking technique, for example, these abdominal muscles are under tremendous strain and accept a good deal of the load from the back muscles. Good hiking technique, by the way, dictates that the knees be bent and the lower back be straight. When the lower back is straight, it is less vulnerable to injury.

The general principle of knee bending to keep the lower back straight also applies to other tasks that impose a heavy load. Lifting, straining, and even prolonged standing should be done with either the knees bent or one foot higher than the other. When weighing an anchor or sweating a line, for example, place one foot on an object that is handy (such as a cabintop or railing).

One final thought: There is nothing wrong with making yourself comfortable. If you are going to be sitting in one place for hours at a time, plan ahead to make the area as comfortable as possible. Any fixed posture takes its toll. But the limit is reached earlier if it is uncomfortable from the beginning!

NOTES

1. The specificity principle even applies to individual aerobic activities. One study, for example, investigated the specificity of swimming training on maximum aerobic power. Fifteen men trained an hour each day, 3 days a week, for 10 weeks. There were also 15 nontraining control subjects. Before and after training, each subject was measured with both treadmill running and swimming. After the 10 weeks of training, there was an 11 percent improvement in aerobic ability as measured by swimming. However, although it was expected that there would be some "transfer" in aerobic ability from swimming to running, there was none at all. The training subjects performed no better than the nontraining controls!

2. For further information concerning either the art or the science of exercise and athletic training: C. E. Klafs and D. D. Arnheim, *Modern Principles of Athletic Training,* 5th ed. (St. Louis: Mosby, 1981), and W. D. McArdle, F. I. Katch, and V. L. Katch, *Exercise Physiology* (Philadelphia: Lea & Febiger, 1981).

3. One of the few people interested in developing an exercise program specifically directed toward the 12-meter racing sailor is James C. Sattel, Director of Rehabilitation Services at the Newport (Rhode Island) Hospital. He has been refining his

program over the years based on surveys of 12-meter crews. At the present time he plans to test a program that includes a tailored PRE regime 3 days per week and a CT regime 5 to 6 days per week.

10

Sleep, Fatigue, and Performance at Sea

Sleep that knits up the ravell'd
sleave of care,
The death of each day's life,
sore labour's bath,
Balm of hurt minds, great
nature's second course,
Chief nourisher of life's feast.

William Shakespeare, *Macbeth*, 1606

It's been a hard day's night,
I should be sleeping like a log.

The Beatles, "A Hard Day's Night," 1964

SLEEP HAS ALWAYS BEEN highly prized at sea and probably always will be. The problem of obtaining enough of it arises from the unique marine environment with its around-the-clock duties, extended time offshore, and limited supply of manpower. In response, sailors have, over the years, developed a number of different watch-keeping systems with the dual purpose of ensuring that the work is shared equitably and that the opportunities for sleep are maximized.

Sleep is only one part of a large, complex human timekeeping system. A complete cycle in the system normally recurs about every 24 hours, forming what is known as a *circadian rhythm* (in Latin, *circa dies,* "about a day"). In addition to sleep, a number of other body functions are nor-

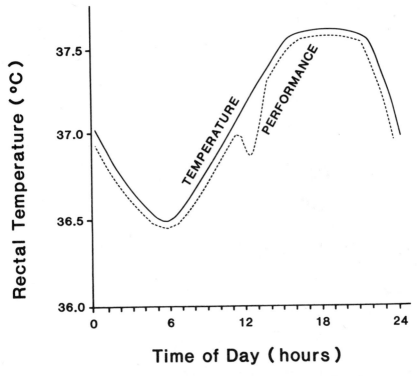

Figure 10.1. *The circadian rhythm of body temperature and performance.*

mally synchronized to this 24-hour circadian system, including body temperature, hormone secretion, salt and water balance, and even some measures of human performance! The advantage of having such a timekeeping system is that it enables the body to predict and prepare for those environmental changes that occur regularly each day. Adaptive responses, which in some cases take several hours to activate, can then be initiated in advance.

Figure 10.1 illustrates the circadian rhythm for sleep, body temperature, and human performance for a typical sailor. At about 0400 or 0500, just before arising in the morning, the body temperature is at its lowest point or "trough." Thereafter it begins to rise, first rapidly, then more slowly throughout the day. In tandem with the rise in body temperature, human performance of a number of tasks also improves during the day. A variety of tests have documented this circadian fluctuation in performance. There have been field studies of hospital workers, factory workers, train engineers, and naval radar operators. In addition, scientists have conducted formal, experimental studies of visual searching and reaction time and a number of so-called psychomotor tests, concentrating on precisely the kinds of skills most crucial to the sailor.[1]

An exception to the gradual improvement in performance throughout the day occurs at about 1300, when there is often a temporary decline (Figure 10.1). This decline, which we have all experienced, is known as the "post-lunch dip," but it occurs whether or not lunch is actually eaten. That is, this temporary decline in performance seems to be a built-in feature of the circadian rhythm. Following the post-lunch dip, temperature and performance again increase in tandem to a maximum level at about 2000. Thereafter, temperature and performance begin to decline. The sailor soon becomes tired, and sleep usually commences between 2300 and 2400. The majority of adults sleep approximately 8 hours, during which time the body temperature continues to decline.

Although the temperature and performance curves mirror one another throughout most of the day, it is a mistake to consider that the rise or fall in body temperature *causes* the increase or decrease in performance. On the contrary, each of the components in the circadian system is independent. Under normal circumstances temperature, performance, and the sleep-wake cycles are synchronized. However, as we will see shortly, if we disrupt the normal circadian rhythm (which is inevitable with many of the watch-keeping systems), we can desynchronize the system, causing the various components to adopt independent rhythms. (See discussion later in this chapter.)

It should now be apparent why the night watches present the greatest opportunity for accident, error, and other misfortune. Most likely the sailor has stood one or more daytime watches and may already have accumulated a certain amount of sleep loss. Fatigue interferes with his performance just as he is approaching the time of day when his performance is normally at its worst—a kind of double whammy.

MANIPULATING THE RHYTHM OF SLEEP

In order to appreciate the degree to which the circadian sleep-wake cycle can be modified, let us examine two situations that all of us face from time to time: jet lag and the "Monday morning blues."

Man's internal time is synchronized with external time by a number of environmental cues or zeitgebers (literally "time givers" in German), which structure the daily, 24-hour routine. Zeitgebers include light and darkness, activity and rest, meal routines, personal interactions, and other social rituals. Sometimes, though, internal and external time get out of sync. For example, if you leave New York at 1900 on a flight to London, you will arrive in London at, say, 0800 local time. But due to the 5-hour time difference, it will be 0300 New York time. Nevertheless, you may be expected to function straightaway at a high level of performance despite the fact that if you were back in New York you would be in the midst of your normal sleep period. If, by 2300 London time, you decide to go to sleep, this will correspond to a late afternoon (1800) nap in New York time. And on awakening the next morning at 0700 London time, you will probably feel as though it were 0200 New York time—and for good reason! Although the sleep-wake cycle resynchronizes in a couple of days, it takes approximately 7 to 10 days for the entire circadian system to resynchronize under optimal circumstances, that is, when time shifts only once and all of the zeitgebers stay in concert. But in addition to its heuristic value, the jet-lag syndrome has a number of practical consequences. It is now common practice to fly all or part of the crew to the vessel, which may be on the other side of the globe. These crew members are often expected to participate immediately in the watch-keeping system of the ship. This is usual procedure on merchant vessels, which invariably sail with a "bare-bones" crew and must fly in replacements. The practice is not unknown to the rest of the sailing community either. If the sailor who is still disoriented from jet lag is now subjected to a continually changing watch-keeping schedule, it is easy to imagine that his circadian rhythm may not straighten itself out for weeks!

Another common example of desynchronization is the Monday morning blues. During the week we normally sleep from 2300 to 0700. What happens if we stay out late on Saturday night and don't retire until 0200? We temporarily *phase delay* our sleep cycle so that we do not arise on Sunday until 1000 or 1100. This usually does not present a significant social problem, since Sunday is an "off" day. The difficulty begins Sunday night when we try to *phase advance* our sleep cycle (i.e., go to sleep earlier), find ourselves unable to, and suffer insomnia. Sleep may not be possible until, say, 0100. Even worse, on arising Monday morning at the usual 0700, it seems like the middle of a sleep period. No wonder Monday morning is often such a dreadful time of the week! Occasionally, this phase delay can be used to advantage, for example, if the sailor needs to stay awake for one night in an overnight race or cruise. Simply staying up late the night before and sleeping late the morning of the race or cruise will phase delay the cycle. The sailor doubtless finds the subsequent night watch more tolerable.

This illustration highlights an important rule concerning manipulation of the sleep-wake cycle: it is much easier to phase delay the cycle (stay awake) for a few hours than it is to phase advance it (retire early).

How do various watch-keeping schedules affect our composite circadian rhythm? There are basically three possibilities: (1) the rhythm remains fundamentally intact, (2) it deteriorates, or (3) it becomes phase shifted by a certain number of hours (as with a time-zone change).

The composite circadian rhythm tends to remain intact to the extent that the new schedule resembles the previous sleep-wake cycle. At least a few hours of sleep taken approximately the same time each night will "anchor" the overall cycle. This is more likely to occur with a "fixed" rather than with a "rotating" schedule.

With rapidly rotating schedules, however, the body usually responds in one of two ways. First, if there are a number of conflicting zeitgebers, the body may say nix and generate its own rhythm, a phenomenon known as *free running*. Free running was first discovered in isolation experiments when subjects were removed from all zeitgebers. Deprived of external cues, the body generates its own circadian rhythm, which, interestingly, has a cycle length of about 25 hours rather than 24! Second, the individual rhythms may undergo *desynchronization,* each going its own way. Although we know very little about the short- or long-term health consequences of either free running or desynchronization, it is doubtful they can be beneficial. One possible deleterious effect of desynchronization appears to be impaired body-temperature regulation. At least in monkeys, desynchronization hinders the ability to withstand cold exposure. It is not yet known whether desynchronization facilitates the development of hypothermia in man.

Phase shifting the circadian rhythm is the most difficult to effect, but in terms of ultimate night-shift performance, it is probably the most desirable. Unfortunately, only two of the watch-keeping schedules to be discussed offer phase shifting as a possibility, and both are three-watch systems.

Before we analyze specific watch-keeping systems, a few additional sleep concepts need to be addressed. First, there is evidence that sleep requirements can be slightly reduced. In one sleep-reduction study, subjects reduced their sleep by 30 minutes every 2 to 4 weeks until it was reduced overall by 1 to 4 hours. In most of the subjects a sleep reduction of 1 to 2 hours occurred without any significant change in either mood or performance. It seems that with training we can learn to sleep more efficiently![2]

Second, research continues to define differences between "morning" and "evening" people. This has potential practical consequences for choosing the most suitable candidates for night shifts. A *circadian-type questionnaire* has also been developed and is currently being tested.

Last, naps are an invaluable source of sleep for the sailor. Although sleep is most refreshing when taken in a single, uninterrupted block, any sleep is worth taking. Some research suggests, however, that naps in the morning are less effective than those taken in the afternoon.

CHOOSING A WATCH-KEEPING SYSTEM

The number of possible watch-keeping systems is virtually limitless. The major determinants are the tasks that need to be performed and the crew that can be carried. These two variables determine the number of watches that can be set. If at all possible, the captain should *not* stand a set watch, since he is already expected (unrealistically) to be at peak efficiency on an around-the-clock basis. Once the number of watches has been decided upon, the choice of a specific watch-keeping schedule largely depends on balancing the need for quality performance with the requirement for an equitable distribution of the unwanted shifts.

One Watch

The most serious limitation in having only one watch is that inevitably there are periods when there is not *any* watch! This is one of the accepted hazards of singlehanded sailing. In the 1972 OSTAR, information on sleeping routine was available for 21 sailors. Five woke hourly, or more often than hourly, all, or nearly all, the time. One of these managed to wake himself every half hour, day and night, for 38 days. Four sailors established a schedule in which they woke less often than every hour. Twelve singlehanders did not establish a sleep-wake schedule, but slept at irregular intervals. Unfortunately the numbers were too small (and there were too many other variables) to establish whether the sleep-wake routine had a recognizable effect on sailing efficiency.[3]

Two Watches

There are at least five two-watch schedules that we can discuss (Figure 10.2). The most popular system (at least with the "if-it-was-good-enough-for-Nelson-it's-good-enough-for-me" crowd) is the traditional "watch and watch" or "4 on, 4 off" (Figure 10.2A). It can be used with or without

(continued on page 218)

Figure 10.2A through J. Watch-keeping schedules.

Figure 10.2A. 4-hour fixed watches.

Day	A	B
	0800-1200	1200-1600
	1600-2000	2000-2400
	2400-0400	0400-0800
Day 1	0800-1200	1200-1600
	1600-2000	2000-2400
	2400-0400	0400-0800
Day 2	0800-1200	1200-1600
	1600-2000	2000-2400
	2400-0400	0400-0800
Day 3	0800-1200	1200-1600
	1600-2000	2000-2400
	2400-0400	0400-0800

Figure 10.2B. 4-hour rotating watches.

Day	A	B
	0800-1200	1200-1600
	1600-1800	1800-2000
	2000-2400	2400-0400
	0400-0800	
Day 1	0800-1200	1200-1600
	1600-1800	1800-2000
	2000-2400	2400-0400
	0400-0800	
Day 2	0800-1200	1200-1600
	1600-1800	1800-2000
	2000-2400	2400-0400
	0400-0800	
Day 3	0800-1200	1200-1600
	1600-1800	1800-2000
	2000-2400	2400-0400
	0400-0800	

Figure 10.2C. Modified traditional system.

Day	A	B
	1000-1400	1400-1800
	1800-2000	2000-2200
	2200-0200	0200-0600
		0600-1000
Day 1	1400-1800	1000-1400
	2000-2200	1800-2000
	0200-0600	2200-0200
		0600-1000
Day 2	1000-1400	0600-1000
	1800-2000	1400-1800
	2200-0200	2000-2200
		0200-0600
Day 3	0600-1000	1000-1400
	1400-1800	1800-2000
	2000-2200	2200-0200
	0200-0600	
		0600-1000

Figure 10.2D. Swedish system.

	A	B
Day 1	0800–1400	
		1400–2000
	2000–2400	
		2400–0400
	0400–0800	
		0800–1400
Day 2	1400–2000	
		2000–2400
	2400–0400	
	0400–0800	
		0800–1400
Day 3	1400–2000	
		2000–2400
	2400–0400	
	0400–0800	

Figure 10.2D. Swedish system.

Figure 10.2E. 5-hour night watches.

	A	B
Day 1	0900–1200	1200–1500
	1500–1900	1900–2300
	2300–0400	0400–0900
	0900–1200	1200–1500
	1500–1900	1900–2300
Day 2	2300–0400	0400–0900
	0900–1200	1200–1500
	1500–1900	1900–2300
	2300–0400	0400–0900
Day 3	0900–1200	1200–1500
	1500–1900	1900–2300
	2300–0400	0400–0900

Figure 10.2E. 5-hour night watches.

	A	B	C
	0800–1200		
		1200–1600	
			1600–2000
	2000–2400		
		2400–0400	
			0400–0800
	0800–1200		
Day 1		1200–1600	
			1600–2000
	2000–2400		
		2400–0400	
			0400–0800
	0800–1200		
Day 2		1200–1600	
			1600–2000
	2000–2400		
		2400–0400	
			0400–0800
	0800–1200		
Day 3		1200–1600	
			1600–2000
	2000–2400		
		2400–0400	
			0400–0800

Figure 10.2F. 4 on/8 off.

	A	B	C
	0900–1200	1200–1500	1500–1800
	1800–2100	2100–2400	
			2400–0300
	0300–0600	0600–0900	0900–1200
Day 1	1200–1500	1500–1800	1800–2100
	2100–2400		
		2400–0300	0300–0600
Day 2	0600–0900	0900–1200	1200–1500
	1500–1800	1800–2100	2100–2400
	2400–0300	0300–0600	0600–0900
Day 3	0900–1200	1200–1500	1500–1800
	1800–2100	2100–2400	
			2400–0300
	0300–0600	0600–0900	

Figure 10.2G. 3 on/6 off.

	A	B	C
		0800–1200	
	1200–1600		
			1600–2000
		2000–2400	
			2400–0400
	0400–0800		
Day 1			0800–1200
		1200–1600	
	1600–2000		
			2000–2400
	2400–0400		
		0400–0800	
Day 2	0800–1200		
			1200–1600
		1600–2000	
	2000–2400		
		2400–0400	
			0400–0800
Day 3		0800–1200	
	1200–1600		
			1600–2000
		2000–2400	
			2400–0400
	0400–0800		

Figure 10.2H. Royal rotating watch system.

	A	B	C
Day 1	0800–1600	1600–2400	2400–0800
Day 2	0800–1600	1600–2400	2400–0800
Day 3	0800–1600	1600–2400	2400–0800

Figure 10.2I. Fixed 8-hour watches.

	A	B	C
	0820–1640	1640–0100	0100–0920
Day 1	0920–1740	1740–0200	0200–1020
Day 2	1020–1840	1840–0300	0300–1120
Day 3	1120–1940	1940–0400	0400–1220

Figure 10.2J. 25-hour day.

(continued from page 213)

the "dogged watch" (1600 to 1800 and 1800 to 2000), depending on whether or not rotation is desired (Figure 10.2*B*). The fixed schedule may have a slight advantage in that it disrupts the circadian cycle less and hence may improve overall performance, particularly on the night shifts. The rotating schedule, however, tends to be more easily accepted. Some sailors become discouraged at the thought of having the same night shift for the entire voyage.

Many sailors will recognize the continuity of their sailing heritage in the following passage from John Masefield's *Sea Life in Nelson's Time*. Although the duties may have changed somewhat, the ebb and flow of the daily routine are essentially the same today as in Nelson's time:

> The day of a man-of-war's man began at midnight, or at four in the morning, according to the alternation of the watches. If he had the middle-watch, from 12 P.M. till 4 A.M., he came on deck at midnight and remained there till 4 A.M., doing any duty which appeared necessary.... The men had but to trim the sails, and be ready for a call.... The remainder of the watch were supposed by the Articles of War to keep awake on pain of death. Some captains and lieutenants allowed those not actually on watch as look-out men to sleep during their night-watches, if the weather was very fine. The act of sleeping during a night watch in the tropics was known as "taking a caulk," because by lying on the plank-seams the sailors' jackets were marked with lines of tar. In those ships aboard which the sailors were expected to keep awake, the boatswain's mates walked round with their starters, or kept buckets of water ready to wake anyone who fell asleep....
>
> A few minutes before eight bells, or 4 A.M., the quarter-masters stole down the after-ladders to call the midshipmen, mates, and lieutenant of the other watch. The boatswain's mates... blew the prolonged, shrill call "All Hands" following it up by a shout of "Starboard (or larboard) Watch Ahoy. Rouse Out There, You Sleepers. Hey. Out or Down Here." At this order, the watch below, who were snugly sleeping in their hammocks, turned out at once without waiting till they were properly awake. When they had turned out they put on their clothes (if they had taken them off) and bustled up on deck with the starters after them.... The men of the other watch, who had kept the deck since midnight, were then allowed to go below to their hammocks.
>
> ...Before 5 A.M. the watch took off their trousers to the thigh, rigged the pumps, got out the scrubbers and buckets, and began to wash the ship down.... At about half-past seven the boatswain's mates went below to the berth-deck and piped "All Hands. Up Hammocks," a pipe which brought up the sleepers and filled the deck with scurrying figures.... By 8 A.M. at a word from the captain the boatswain piped to breakfast, eight bells was struck upon the ship's bell, and nearly every man except the helmsman, lookout men, and officers on duty, slipped down to breakfast. Half-an-hour was allowed for this meal on weekdays. At half-past eight the watch was

called, and those who had slept from 4 till 7:30 A.M. came upon deck...
employed in the work of the ship, in the rigging, or about the guns, doing
the never-finished duties of sailormen.

...Dinner generally took about half-an-hour, from twelve till half-past.
It was a merry meal, eaten cheerily, with a great buzz of talk all along the
gun deck. At half-past twelve there came a great clink of cans and banging
of tin plates on the tables. The fifer took his flute to the main or upper
deck, where the master's mate stood by the tub to dispense sea ambrosia
to the ship's company.... Grog time was the one happy hour of the day.
With grog and an occasional battle a sailor was often almost contented.

At half-past one o'clock, when the last oozings of the black jack had been
drained, the watch on deck was called to duty. The watch below were
sometimes allowed to keep below, to sleep if they could.... At 4 P.M. the
boatswain piped to supper, which lasted half-an-hour, and was made pleas-
ant by the second serving out of grog. Shortly after supper, but before sunset,
the drummer beat to quarters. All hands had to repair to their stations.

...At eight o'clock the first night-watch was called and set, and the watch
below went down to their hammocks until midnight. The lights were ex-
tinguished, or covered over, so that they would not show from a distance....

The watch and watch system, four hours on and four hours off, with
the four hours off constantly broken in upon by the ship's routine, was severe
and harassing. It meant that the sailor had but four hours of sleep one night,
and a bare seven hours the night following. The little naps they managed
to take in the forenoons and afternoons were hardly worth mentioning; they
were too uncertain, too liable to interruption. Even in their watches below
at night they were liable to be called on deck to tack, to wear, to shorten
sail, or to go to their stations. Once a month, at least, they were drummed
up to general quarters in the middle of their dreams.[4]

There is nothing sacrosanct about the timing of the watches. Tradition
would have us continue to rotate our 4-hour shifts on a 4-8-12-4-8-12
schedule—and there are advantages. For instance, the traditional mealtimes
for breakfast (0800), lunch (1200), and dinner (1800) correspond to changes
of the watch (Figure 10.2B). This allows a single preparation for both the
oncoming as well as the off-going watches. The disadvantage, however,
is that the first of the three watches during which the sailor is expected
to sleep (2000 to 2400) contains at least 3 hours (2000 to 2300) in which
sleep is difficult to obtain, since that would require him to phase advance
his cycle. A "modified traditional" system (Figure 10.2C) attempts to
alleviate this problem by shifting all of the watches 2 hours. Every other
night the sailor should be able to get 7 to 8 hours of sleep.

An increasingly popular schedule for both cruising and racing sailors
is the so-called Swedish system (Figure 10.2D). It retains three late 4-hour
watches but combines the three daytime watches into two 6-hour shifts,
in a conscious attempt to provide at least one long, uninterrupted period
during the day to catch up on lost sleep. Unfortunately, there are

unavoidable problems with daytime sleep. Unless the sleeping quarters are "far from the madding crowd," daytime noises make sleep difficult. Also, sleep taken during the day after a night shift is invariably "lighter" and shorter than nighttime sleep. The sailor may unwittingly exacerbate the situation by getting up prematurely rather than lying in bed with the chance of going back to sleep.

An altogether different approach would be to lengthen the night watch instead of shortening it! If the two night watches were 5 hours instead of 4, both watches could theoretically get 5 hours of relatively "prime-time" sleep each night. The remainder of the day could be divided into two 3-hour and two 4-hour watches (Figure 10.2*E*). This kind of a watch-keeping schedule would only be feasible if the other fatigue-producing factors were either mild or absent. One disadvantage of the system is that it is nonrotational, although that could be used to advantage if the crew were composed of an equal number of "morning" and "evening" types.

Three Watches

The "4 on, 8 off" (Figure 10.2*F*) is the logical extension of the traditional "watch and watch" system. The only difference is that the former is a fixed system, and there is no easy way to rotate the watches. Therefore, one of the watches is stuck with the disagreeable 0400 to 0800 tour of duty for the duration of the voyage or until the rotation is altered. In general, it takes a couple of weeks to adjust to a fixed night watch. Unless there is an overriding necessity, fixed shifts should be allowed to run for at least 3 or 4 weeks at a time.

Although the "4 on, 8 off" may be "unfair," the advantage of the schedule (as with any fixed schedule) is that it permits the crew member to organize his life and get used to working nights. Sleep can then be taken the same time or times each day.

If "fairness" is an overriding concern, then the "3 on, 6 off" might be worth considering (Figure 10.2*G*). It rotates by phase delaying 3 hours each day if the sailor puts off most of his sleep until after he has worked two consecutive shifts. It is doubtful whether any sailor would continue to phase delay around the clock. Rather, after 3 days of phase delaying, most sailors try to phase advance on the fourth day. Also, if the sailor chooses to split his sleep in two, there is a tendency for the schedule to degenerate into 18-hour "days." This places a severe strain on the circadian cycle and promotes a free-running behavior.

The Royal Navy has used a watch system that at first glance looks almost random (Figure 10.2*H*). Actually, it provides a 3-day cycle during which each of the three watches works every 4-hour shift one time. It does leave considerable time periods during the day to catch up on lost sleep.

Probably the best overall three-watch schedule is that of fixed 8-hour shifts. Most merchant ships in the United States and England use this system. It has all of the advantages of a fixed system. In addition, since sleep can be taken in one 8-hour block (either before or after work), the entire circadian cycle may be shifted (Figure 10.2*I*). However, it may take a couple of weeks to shift the cycle, and a number of experiments have shown that even after a prolonged stint on the night shift, not all of the rhythms are perfectly shifted. The explanation is that (except on a submarine) it is impossible to shift *all* of the zeitgebers. In fact, this is a major complaint of people who are "permanently" on the night shift. Many opportunities, such as those for social interaction, are unavailable on this shift. Another consideration is that to make this shift work, there must be enough crew members assigned to each watch so that various jobs can be rotated. Otherwise, an 8-hour shift is much too fatiguing for most onboard tasks.

One schedule offers the best of both worlds—the improved performance at night of the fixed, long watches and the equitable distribution of unpleasant watches inherent in a rotating system—the "25-hour" day (Figure 10.2*J*). As we have seen, a free-running rhythm is usually 25 hours long, and phase delaying by 1 hour is well within the capabilities of the human circadian system. The simplest way to achieve this is to have shifts of 8 hours and 20 minutes in length (with off-watch periods of 16 hours and 40 minutes). Although Nelson would turn over in his grave, this system has a lot to recommend it. To date, no one in the maritime community has accepted the challenge to try it.[5]

FATIGUE

Fatigue is the archenemy of the mariner since it undermines both his vigilance and his performance. In the process it severely jeopardizes the safety of the vessel and crew. Many experienced sailors can doubtless recall episodes in which fatigue produced disastrous or near disastrous results: the familiar channel light that for no apparent reason was misinterpreted or the foolish navigational error in home waters that threatened the entire voyage. The high rate of accidents among trawlermen has been attributed to their fatigue-producing schedule.

What is fatigue and how is it capable of transforming the most able-bodied seaman into a dangerous, muddleheaded bumpkin? The term *fatigue* is derived from the Latin *fatigare,* meaning "to waste away." Many scientific and technical disciplines make use of the term in this sense to denote a change in some property from a stronger to a weaker state. To the metallurgist, fatigue implies a progressive deterioration in the strength of the metal associated with crystalline changes in its structure resulting from repeated stresses. To the exercise physiologist, fatigue implies a decrease in muscle strength associated with depleted energy reserves and an increase in breakdown products such as lactic acid. For the psychologist, fatigue describes a mental state characterized by decreased motivation, an elevated threshold for stimuli, and a decrease in accuracy and speed in solving problems or carrying out psychomotor tasks. We can operationally define fatigue as *a deterioration in the capacity to maintain a state of vigilance and an accompanying decline in the ability to think and act effectively.*

The effects of fatigue can be roughly divided into two phases. During the *first phase of fatigue,* the sailor experiences a feeling of excessive tiredness and a reluctance to do what needs to be done—such as reefing, tidying up, taking a bearing, or doing chart work. The expression "The time to reef is when you first think about it" was formulated for just such moments when the sailor is looking for some excuse to avoid the task at hand. At first this reluctance may be subtle (and is often misinterpreted), but within a short period of time the weariness and lassitude of the crew become manifest. William F. Buckley, Jr., describes just such a state after he and his crew spent more than a day battling a mid-Atlantic storm. This included a missed night's sleep: "It was about 7:00 P.M. that I became creepingly aware that the crew was demoralized. No one would eat. The dishes were piled up from the last three meals. There was no conversation, no unnecessary motion."[6]

Poor concentration and simple forgetfulness are also early signs of fatigue. The 1972 OSTAR produced the following example:

> After a trip up the mast to repair a broken shroud, one singlehander found that he would go below to fetch something and then forget what he had gone for. The next day he "tried to put a saucepan away in the cutlery drawer," and again "made a pot of tea this morning which I had been looking forward to—left it for 15 minutes to draw, having promptly forgotten about it, not distracted by any other important duty." After a couple of days his function returned to its usual high level of efficiency.[7]

Activities like cooking that require both coordination and concentration frequently show up minor errors in performance. Although the results of such errors are usually more humorous than dangerous, they should serve to alert the sailor that he is experiencing fatigue. Probably the most complex task the sailor must perform is navigation, and it abounds with possibilities for error. There are, after all, so many places for errors to creep in and go undetected: sightings or bearings to be misobserved, times to be inaccurately taken, tables to be misread, and a myriad of potential calculation errors. Sir Francis Chichester reported such an experience in *Alone Across the Atlantic:*

> When I came to plot the night's doings on the chart I found I had made a most stupid blunder the night before in my plotting. There were two charts on the chart table. The top one on which I was plotting had its left-hand margin turned down to make it fit on the chart table. The edge of the chart below was showing on the left and I had measured my distance off the coast from its latitude scale which was less than half the scale of the chart above. (This was all by candle light.) Therefore instead of being 20 miles from land I must have been only 8 off and when I tacked only 3. Therefore, had I gone into a deep sleep for two hours I might have had a rude awakening.[8]

In the 1972 OSTAR, no other category of error showed up as frequently as navigational error, often attributable to fatigue.

The *second phase of fatigue* is essentially a continuation of the first. Vigilance is even more impaired than before. Tiredness and uncontrollable sleepiness now come in waves and may cause lapses into brief periods of sleep, which may make it difficult for the sailor to tell whether he is awake or asleep. " 'My mind was completely separated from my body,' said one competitor [in the 1972 OSTAR]. 'I just used my body to get around the boat. Eventually there was no difference between sleeping and waking. You went about in a kind of sleep-wake.' "[9]

The sailor may now begin to display atypical emotional reactions. Changes in personality may surface, such as unusual irritability or unaccustomed passivity. With extreme degrees of fatigue, there may be inappropriate and uncontrollable laughter or crying.

At this point, the stress of fatigue is beginning to disrupt the basic functioning of the brain. The simplest tasks can be accomplished only with great difficulty and are fraught with errors. Complex tasks are well beyond the capabilities of the sailor. Most dangerous of all, the senses, upon which we ultimately depend for the information with which to make decisions, become unreliable. The sailor may begin to experience illusions (misinterpretations of what is seen or heard) or even frank hallucinations (visual or auditory images of nonexistent objects). Illusions and hallucinations are explored in greater depth in Chapter 11. It is sufficient to note that unless something is done to rectify the situation, the crew and vessel are in serious jeopardy.

FATIGUE AND PERFORMANCE

What factors produce fatigue and/or otherwise impair the sailor's performance? Clearly the most important is the lack of *sleep*. The earliest signs of fatigue may surface when the sailor has incurred a sleep debt of only 5 hours. Simple monitoring tasks are particularly sensitive since there is nothing to do but wait and watch—and while waiting the sailor may periodically doze off! It should be noted that a normal night's sleep does not fully compensate for a night without sleep. Also, sailors should realize that it takes 5 to 7 minutes after awakening to function at peak efficiency. If the need for prompt action is anticipated, it may be better to stay awake.

Even in the absence of sleep loss, *constant vigilance* of any kind is an extremely demanding task. In an unbroken period of monitoring (such as looking for a light or listening for a horn), the likelihood of detecting the signal starts to decline almost as soon as the sailor begins the task! The decrease of vigilance is easily demonstrated after 20 minutes. This is known to psychologists as the vigilance-decrement phenomenon. For example, one study of a simulated continuous sonar watch demonstrated that the extent of the decline may be considerable. Even in the daytime watches, the rate deteriorated by 20 percent over the 4-hour period with most of the deterioration in the early part of the watch. The important point is whether or not the task is continuous. It is well documented that if another task or a rest period breaks up a vigilance-monitoring period, that performance decline can be reduced considerably. Thus, there is a rationale for rotating jobs within a watch period. But, variation and decline in performance can never be entirely eliminated. It is, to some extent, a function of *la condition humaine* and is beyond our control.

As we have seen, performance varies throughout the day in a rhythmic 24-hour cycle, known as the circadian performance rhythm (Figure 10.1). Recent studies have also demonstrated additional, shorter performance rhythms (technically known as ultradian rhythms) with a frequency range of 10 to 20 cycles per day; that is, performance on certain tasks varies about every 100 minutes or so. Although we cannot currently alter these fluctuations in performance, we should at least be aware of them.[10]

The fact that performance on purely motor tasks, such as steering, varies in a predictable fashion is well known. Usually it takes 5 to 10 minutes at the helm to "get into the groove." Experienced sailors confirm that after about another half-hour their ability to keep a heading begins to decline, perhaps somewhat more slowly with more experienced sailors. Two hours at the helm is just about the limit in good conditions; otherwise, shorter schedules are in order.

OTHER FACTORS THAT AFFECT PERFORMANCE

Obviously the *physical condition* of the sailor affects his overall performance. This includes his general health as well as the exercise schedule he maintains. The *nutritional status* of the sailor is not a major factor over the short term, unless he has previously been nutritionally deprived. The diagnosis of hypoglycemia has become fashionable in American culture, which seems to put a label on every minor indisposition. Thus it is overworked. Most people who claim to have hypoglycemia do not have it. We are able to fast for long periods of time without becoming hypoglycemic. Nevertheless, there is incontrovertible evidence that hunger contributes to the development of fatigue and that a good meal often has a salubrious effect. Whether or not the effect is psychological is unknown and of little importance.

Alcohol and the *depressant drugs* exacerbate fatigue and impair performance. Their effect is roughly additive with any of the other causes listed here. Drugs that have a depressant effect include sleeping pills, tranquilizers and antidepressants, many of the seasickness medications (see Chapter 1), and most of the cold preparations. Alcohol occupies a special place in the hearts and minds of sailors. Many would no more leave the dock without their six-pack than they would without their sails or rudder. This relationship between man and his alcohol has a long historic precedent (see Chapter 5), yet alcohol is the proximate cause for numerous marine accidents each year and a contributing factor in many others. One study showed that 47 percent of adults who drowned had evidence of alcohol in their blood. Clearly, if alcohol were just being introduced, the boating community would probably ban it—not to mention the FDA! Nevertheless, alcohol is here to stay, and we are better off understanding its effects than merely railing against its consequences.

Alcohol may be detected in the blood within 5 minutes after ingestion, and the maximum concentration is reached within 30 to 90 minutes. The ingestion of fatty foods and milk impedes its absorption, whereas water facilitates it. The metabolism of alcohol is unlike most other drugs, which are eliminated according to their "half life"; that is, in a given period of time the level of the drug is reduced by half, then by half again, and so on. The metabolism of alcohol proceeds at a constant rate regardless of the concentration. A 150-pound (70-kilogram) person metabolizes 70 to 100 grams of alcohol per hour. This is equivalent to ⅔ to 1 ounce (20 to 30 milliliters) of 90 proof spirits *or* 8 to 12 ounces of beer (235 to 355 milliliters).

We are all aware that alcohol adversely affects motor performance, including standing posture, speech, and highly organized or complex motor skills. The movements not only are slower than normal but also are more inaccurate and random in character. The same disintegration is true of eye movements. Thus, relatively mild intoxication impairs the performance of any skilled task that requires rapid visual perception. Alcohol also impairs the efficiency of mental function such as concentrating, remembering, making judgments, and solving problems. In sum, alcohol adversely affects virtually all aspects of performance. Finally, male crew members "under the influence" should consider, as they dangle from the backstay to relieve themselves, that the Latin term *urinator* described one who was a diver!

Environmental factors also play a role in limiting performance. Heavy-weather sailing is known to reduce endurance and accelerate fatigue. So does anything that increases the general discomfort of the sailor—uncomfortable seats, cramped quarters, and wet clothing, for example. Extreme cold or warm weather also impairs performance.

All of these factors need to be taken into consideration when planning a watch-keeping schedule.

NOTES

1. To complicate matters, however, there is some evidence that pure memory tasks may follow a different circadian rhythm, which has a peak in the early morning and a trough in the late afternoon/early evening—exactly the opposite of the psychomotor curve. For the sailor, chart work is the most memory-loaded task. The above evidence would suggest that the morning is the optimal time to do the most complex navigational calculations. Many sailors have already discovered this fact. More research is needed in this area.

2. L. C. Johnson, "On Varying Work/Sleep Schedules: Issues and Perspectives As Seen by a Sleep Researcher," in *Biological Rhythms, Sleep and Shift Work,* edited by L. C. Johnson, W. P. Colquhoun, D. I. Tepas, and M. J. Colligan (New York: SP Medical and Scientific Books, 1981), pp. 335-346.

3. Glin Bennet, "Medical and Psychological Problems in the 1972 Single-

handed Transatlantic Yacht Race," *Lancet* 2 (1973): 747-754. Dr. Bennet has thoroughly studied the "face of fatigue" in sailors who are undoubtedly the most vulnerable—the singlehanded ocean racers. He evaluated the performance of 34 of the 55 competitors in the 1972 Observer's Singlehanded Transatlantic Race (OSTAR). The competitors kept a daily record of activity, progress, and subjective state, noting in particular any general medical problems or difficulty with sleep.

4. John Masefield, *Sea Life in Nelson's Time* (New York: Macmillan, 1925), pp. 185-193.

5. Dr. Elliot D. Weitzman, neurologist and sleep researcher, proposed a 25-hour watch system to the U.S. Navy for its submarine schedules some years ago. Despite the fact that in such an environment it could be implemented with ease and might solve the rotational watch problems, "the line commanders and naval officers did not appreciate its value!" (Letter, December 14, 1982).

6. William F. Buckley, Jr., *Airborne* (New York: Macmillan, 1976), p. 74.

7. Glin Bennet, "The Tired Sailor," *Yachting Monthly,* September 1973, pp. 1393-1399.

8. Francis Chichester, *Alone Across the Atlantic* (London: Allen & Unwin, and New York: McKay, 1961), p. 158.

9. Bennet, "Medical and Psychological Problems," p. 5.

10. The biological rhythms discussed in this chapter have nothing whatsoever to do with the totally discredited concept of "biorhythms." Biorhythm proponents argue that all human behavior is influenced by three cycles (physical, emotional, and intellectual), which begin at the moment of birth and continue throughout life, affecting performance. Biorhythms have as much validity as palmistry, phrenology, and astrology!

11

Sailing Psychology

*The sea won't tolerate the inept or
pretentious for long. The measure of
a man, whether he is an unranked seaman
or an ex-admiral of the blue—his
hopes and fears, the fiber of his
temper, facets of character that might
otherwise remain hidden all of his life
behind a web of status and sophisti-
cation—are soon known on a long
small-ship voyage.*

Charles A. Borden, *Sea Quest,* 1967

EVERYONE WHO GOES DOWN to the sea in ships has his own set of goals
and expectations. For some sailors it is the personal challenge of
making a successful passage across a bay or around the world. Other sailors
enjoy the organized chaos of sailboat racing; some even revel in the tense
give-and-take of the protest meeting! Still others prefer the sense of solitude
and withdrawal from the hurly-burly of modern society—Walden Pond
on a larger scale.

In addition to goals and expectations, we each carry aboard our own
mental and emotional "baggage"; that is, our own style of decision making, of dealing with discomfort (on occasion even adversity), of interact-
ing with others, and of simply amusing ourselves. This psychological reper-
toire, of course, stamps us as individuals.

Since we are all unique, it is difficult to *predict* how each of us would respond to the variety of stressful situations we can encounter at sea. It would be helpful, for example, if we could predict which sailors are not psychologically "cut out" for long-distance, singlehanded sailing; or whether a particular sailor will "fit in" as a crew member. Nevertheless, although the discipline of psychology cannot yet offer us the means and capacity to make reliable predictions, it has identified *patterns of behavior* and has redefined the *limits of normality* in a number of situations of importance to the sailor. Sometimes the results have been surprising—as in the case of isolation and the singlehanded sailor.

SINGLEHANDED SAILING

The singlehanded sailor must face a staggering array of psychological challenges. Isolation, lack of sleep, physical discomfort, and a multitude of other stresses conspire to reduce an otherwise highly efficient sailor to a dangerously inefficient one. A few sailors—the lone voyagers—appear to thrive on the solitude that most of us would find unbearable. Clearly, they are a rare breed, endowed with an unusual psychological makeup. For the rest of us, long-range singlehanding is an occasional experience. It may be planned (a solitary cruise or solo race) or unplanned (lack of crew or shipwreck). In either case, it behooves us to appreciate the psychological hazards that are involved. These hazards are represented by the three S's: *sensory deprivation, sleep loss,* and *stress.*

Although solitude or isolation can be intensely enjoyable at times, it can also be oppressive and highly dangerous. In a remarkable account of his experience in solitary confinement, Christopher Burney made the following observation: "Variety is not the spice of life; it is the very stuff of it."[1] Although as sailors we are not likely to encounter situations as extreme as solitary confinement, monotony, boredom, and a lack of varied sensory stimuli are important and enduring problems aboard ship.

One of the first shipboard concerns to be addressed systematically was that of boredom and job-related monotony. In studies for the Royal Air Force during World War II, N. H. Mackworth investigated the phenomenon that radar operators on antisubmarine patrol frequently failed to detect as many U-boats as were known to be operating in the area. The radar operators usually worked in isolation, watching a radar screen for hours at a time. Mackworth developed an analogous laboratory model and found that performance in any prolonged vigilance task (such as a radar operator or lookout performs) begins to decline within 20 minutes. As a result of this and subsequent confirmatory research, the typical tour of duty for such personnel has generally been shortened. An important corollary implication of this study is that if the sailor expects to function at his best, he should be exposed to a varied and variable sensory environment.

Following Mackworth's investigations, interest in brainwashing, aroused during the Korean war, motivated psychologists at McGill University (and later elsewhere) to explore the effects of reducing the overall level of sensory stimulation. These studies, collectively known as sensory-deprivation experiments, have been conducted in a number of ways. First, the absolute amount of stimuli that reaches a subject may be reduced, producing true *sensory deprivation.* This was initially accomplished by placing the subject in a totally dark, soundproofed room with gloves and arm bandages to reduce the tactile (touch) stimulation. The water-immersion technique that Len Deighton popularized in *The Ipcress File* produces the same results. Although this degree of sensory deprivation does not occur at sea, visual deprivation is a common occurrence for anyone (including sailors) who must stare off into the uniform blackness of space for long periods of time. This hazard is well known to long-distance truck drivers and aviators. After many hours, they may begin to experience illusions (misinterpretations of something that is seen, heard, or felt, for example) or hallucinations (images of nonexistent objects) as a result of the visual deprivation. The nature of the illusions and hallucinations is discussed shortly.

Second, the absolute amount of stimulation may be kept constant, but the variability may be reduced. This is referred to as *perceptual deprivation* and is simulated in the laboratory by special goggles that admit only diffuse, unpatterned light and earphones that transmit meaningless sounds. The effects of perceptual deprivation are similar to those of sensory deprivation.[2] For the sailor, the unchanging visual pattern of the sea, the monotonous sound of the wind in the rigging, and the steady noise of the waves ensures that at least some degree of perceptual deprivation can be expected on every blue-water cruise.

There are two additional situations capable of wreaking havoc with the human psyche: *immobilization* and *social isolation.* Immobilization is rarely a problem for the sailor, but social isolation certainly is. Every singlehanded sailor must deal in one way or another with social isolation. Its symptoms are virtually identical with those of sensory or perceptual deprivation.

What are the symptoms of which the sailor should be cognizant? Often there is an early decline in performance, including both fine and gross motor skills. Perception may also be affected with objects appearing larger or smaller than normal, or straight lines seeming to be curved. Some sailors develop an impaired ability to concentrate and maintain a train of thought. The perception of time passage may be grossly distorted. An alteration in mood is also common and on occasion an oscillation between irritability and euphoria, which may appear childish. Sensory-deprived subjects are said to be more susceptible to persuasion (brainwashing).

The most characteristic symptoms, however, are illusions and hallucinations. Dr. Glin Bennet has written extensively on the psychological phenomena of singlehanded sailors. In his study of the 1972 OSTAR, he examined the type and frequency of perceptual disturbances among the racers. Half of the competitors who completed daily records experienced one or more illusions or hallucinations! Auditory sensations were the most common, followed by visual, olfactory (smell), and spatial *(déjà vu)*. One singlehanded sailor whom Dr. Bennet studied had the following experience after a long stint at the helm:

> He saw his father-in-law at the top of the mast. They were aware of one another's presence, and the experience was in no way alarming. At the top of the mast there is a metal radar reflector, a box-like structure 12 in. (30 cm.) or so across. A short time later the same evening he looked down into the cabin and saw his wife, then his mother, then his daughter lying on the bunk where a sleeping bag was stretched out. Later again he was up at the bows changing a sail and saw in the water by the bows a large flat fish like a ray—very unlikely off the east coast of England—which was probably a misinterpretation of the boat's bow wave....

On occasion, the visual hallucinations may be quite complex, as the following case demonstrates:

> The sailor was lying below on his bunk when he heard someone on deck putting the boat about on the other tack. He stirred himself to go up and investigate, but as he went up on deck an unidentified man passed him coming down into the cabin. On deck he found that the boat had indeed been put about properly and that everything was in order. The process was repeated several times. As the sailor went up the man came down; when the sailor came down the man went up. But the man was not recognized.[3]

As the first example demonstrates, it is often difficult to distinguish illusions from hallucinations and even from dreams, daydreams, images, or fantasies. For this reason, psychologists often refer to all of these visual experiences as *reported visual sensations*. Often (but not invariably) illusions precede hallucinations, and less complex hallucinations (dots, lines, patterns) precede more complex hallucinations (such as animals or people).

Auditory illusions and hallucinations are even more common than visual ones. During a gale, one of the OSTAR racers felt that voices in the rigging were calling "Bill, Bill," in a high-pitched voice. During the same gale, another sailor reported, "Someone knocked on the side deck as if asking to come in. I was petrified."

Vito Dumas, a veteran singlehanded sailor, once overheard the following conversation coming from the forward locker of his boat while sailing from France to South America:[4]

> "Listen," began a voice with a strong Spanish accent, "I'm going to look for something to eat."
> "Shut up; he'll hear you."
> "No, he won't."

At the time, Dumas was not able to leave the helm, but later, when he had the time to investigate, he realized that no one could possibly be stowed away in his forward locker. Even so, the voices were so lifelike that he assumed that people had been on board and that they must have swum ashore (highly improbable).

One widely quoted, complex visual and auditory hallucination was that of Joshua Slocum, the doyen of solo voyagers. His encounter with "the pilot of the *Pinta*" is a classic nautical tale. However, Slocum may have been delirious for reasons other than sensory deprivation (perhaps a toxic reaction, as he suggests), so his case is not a "pure" example:

> Alas! by night-time I was doubled up with cramps. The wind, which was already a smart breeze, was increasing somewhat, with a heavy sky to the sou'west.... I went below, and threw myself upon the cabin floor in great pain. How long I lay there I could not tell, for I became delirious. When I came to, as I thought, from my swoon, I realized the sloop was plunging into a heavy sea, and looking out of the companionway, to my amazement I saw a tall man at the helm. His rigid hand, grasping the spokes of the wheel, held them as in a vise. One may imagine my astonishment. His rig was that of a foreign sailor, and the large red cap he wore was cockbilled over his left ear, and all was set off with shaggy black whiskers. He would have been taken for a pirate in any part of the world. While I gazed upon his threatening aspect I forgot the storm, and wondered if he had come to cut my throat. This he seemed to divine. "Senor," said he, doffing his cap, "I have come to do you no harm." And a smile, the faintest in the world, but still a smile, played on his face, which seemed not unkind when he spoke. "I have come to do you no harm. I have sailed free," he said, "but was never worse than a *contrabandista*. I am one of Columbus's crew," he continued. "I am the pilot of the *Pinta* come to aid you. Lie quiet, senor captain," he added, "and I will guide your ship to-night. You have a *calentura,* but you will be all right to-morrow." I thought what a very devil he

was to carry sail. Again, as if he read my mind, he exclaimed: "Yonder is the *Pinta* ahead; we must overtake her. Give her sail; give her sail! *Vale, vale, muy vale!* " Biting off a large quid of black twist, he said: "You did wrong, captain, to mix cheese with plums. White cheese is never safe unless you know whence it comes. *Quien sabe,* it may have been from *leche de Capra* and becoming capricious.[5]

Any of the other senses may also be involved in sensory-deprivation experiences. Some sailors have reported the feeling of being touched or struck on the arm, whereas others sensed that another body was beside them in their bunk. Still other sailors have reported the smell of cooking or freshly brewed coffee—olfactory hallucinations. *Déjà vu* phenomena, the feeling of having been there before, have also been described.

One OSTAR racer had "this strong feeling of locality—in this case for where I have been becalmed for close on 24 hours. I keep thinking of it as a place I have been to before and can almost picture it." A few days later, "I still have this preoccupation with place, to the extent that if I did not have a compass it would be very easy to become unbalanced about it. It is as though the time and weather conditions constituted a locality."[6]

What can the sailor do to combat the effects of sensory deprivation? Dr. David Lewis has experienced numerous hallucinations on his solo voyages and offers the following suggestion:

When I was very tired, and had spent numerous hours at the helm in winds too light for the vane, I sometimes heard voices.... Hallucinations seem to occur only when solitude and fatigue are accompanied by monotonous occupations.... I would think that varying tasks demanding physical and/or mental effort would be valuable in preserving emotional stability.[7]

Indeed, there is evidence from experimental psychology that *physical* exercise reduces the effects of sensory deprivation. *Mental* exercises are not as helpful and are more difficult to sustain.

The consequences of *sleep loss* have been discussed in Chapter 10. Many of the effects such as mood changes and a decline in performance are similar to those of sensory deprivation. The illusions and hallucinations that occur with sleep loss are indistinguishable from those due to sensory deprivation. In fact, since both hazards frequently occur simultaneously when singlehanded sailing, it is often difficult to place the blame accurately. A typical example would be the singlehanded sailor who is engaged at the helm for hours on end, attempting to claw off a lee shore. If he begins to hallucinate, is it due to his sleep loss? Or is it due to the accumulated solitude of weeks alone at sea? Unlike in the laboratory, it is often impossible to separate the effects of sleep loss from those of sensory deprivation at sea.

The final *S* with which the sailor must cope is *stress,* in its 1,001 nautical forms: being becalmed, battling a storm for 72 hours, avoiding a lee shore, gear failure, and so on. The sailor's underlying personality structure determines, to a great degree, what is stressful to him and how well he can deal with each particular stressful situation. (For individual reactions to highly stressful situations, see "The Psychology of Disaster" later in this chapter.)

If the psychological stresses are severe enough and continue long enough, they may produce a full-blown nervous (psychotic) breakdown. There is some evidence, and it is logical, that these stress-induced breakdowns are more likely to occur in people who have susceptible personalities, especially in those who have suffered nervous breakdowns previously. It seems prudent to suggest that since the psychological stress on the singlehander is so intense, anyone who has had a previous breakdown should forgo singlehanded sailing. But even in the absence of a prior psychiatric disorder, severe environmental stress may produce a psychotic reaction. The best-documented case is that of Donald Crowhurst, a contestant in the 1968 *Sunday Times* around-the-world, singlehanded race. N. Tomalin and R. Hall's *The Strange Last Voyage of Donald Crowhurst* is an extraordinary and disturbing account of the unremitting disintegration of a human psyche. The story is unique because of the extensive documentation available, including logbook writings, tape recordings, and even film.

From the beginning, there were significant psychological stresses: a failing business, tremendous publicity, serious self-doubt, and an ill-prepared and untested boat that was beset with problems. After only 2 weeks at sea Crowhurst realized that the boat would never withstand an around-the-world voyage. At this point he decided to execute an elaborate deception—a fabricated circumnavigation complete with bogus sightings, phony log entries, and faked messages. All the while he was waiting off the east coast of South America for the proper moment to "reenter" the race.

The nervous breakdown occurred over a 1-week period. The apparent cause of the breakdown was the sinking of his nearest rival. He had no means of escaping the hero's welcome that awaited him, and the attendant public scrutiny. Crowhurst harbored suspicions that his deception might be discovered. Prior to the breakdown he was able to sail and navigate with adequate precision, but once his grasp on reality began to loosen, he allowed the boat to drift aimlessly.

His writing, now voluminous, became increasingly cosmic and bizarre:

Mathematicians and engineers used to the techniques of system analysis will skim through my complete work in less than an hour. At the end of that time problems that have beset humanity for thousands of years will have been solved for them. Aspects I have no need to mention will tumble into place, and the distressing struggles of man to reach an understanding of the driving forces between God, Man, and the physical universe [will be over].

He became obsessed with the idea of life as a *game.*

During his lifetime, each man plays cosmic chess against the Devil. Each man can decide for himself who has won. The moves of the game are all well-known. It is a difficult game to follow who is winning the game because God is playing with one set of rules, and the Devil with the other exactly opposite set of rules.

On July 1, the day of his death (and the 243rd day of his voyage), he sat down to set the record straight. His last entries were individually timed, and the final two entries were directed to God, since the next "move" was up to him:

```
11   15   00   It is the end of my
                my game the truth
                has been revealed and it will
                be done as my family require me
                to do it
11   17   00   It is the time for your
                move to begin
                I have not need to prolong
                the game
                It has been a good game that
                must be ended at the
                I will play this game when
                I choose I will resign the
                game 11 20 40 There is
                no reason for harmful[8]
```

At approximately 11 20 40, Donald Crowhurst walked off the boat to merge with the Atlantic Ocean and the universe. The boat, with all of his logs, tape recordings, and home movies, was found 10 days later, floating peacefully, undisturbed.

Should the story of Donald Crowhurst cause concern for singlehanders, or is his a special case? Certainly it is special in the sense that it is so well documented. Most singlehanders who perish do not leave behind such a copious record. Little, however, sets him apart psychologically. He did not suffer from a prior psychiatric disorder, and he never had a previous psychotic breakdown.[9] His symptoms, moreover, are entirely unlike those of sensory deprivation or sleep loss, although it is possible that either may have been contributory. We are forced to conclude that he suffered a stress-induced psychosis.

SAILING CREWS AND SMALL-GROUP BEHAVIOR

It is logical to assume that there are fewer psychological hazards for the small, isolated group, such as a sailing crew, than for the singlehanded sailor. Indeed, the presence of at least one other person does significantly "enrich" the environment. Sailing crew members, for example, experience far fewer episodes of hallucinations, illusions, and other grossly abnormal sensations than do isolated individuals.

But small groups are not without their own stresses. Laboratory experiments of groups in isolation, studies of isolated duty stations in polar regions, accounts of sea voyages and disasters, submarine service, experiences with man-in-space and man-beneath-the-sea all provide examples. Some of the problems of crew behavior can be anticipated and avoided, whereas others can often be successfully defused. The first requirement is to recognize the stresses that the crew is likely to experience.

There are three major stresses: (1) when confined, even the most enriched environment has a tendency to become boring and monotonous; (2) many of the usual sources of gratification and release are no longer available to the crew; and (3) crew members are forced to interact socially in crowded and otherwise unfavorable conditions. The interdependence of crew members blocks many overt means of expressing frustration. After all, a crew member can ill afford to alienate the remainder of the crew.

The degree of stress also depends on the size of the group, its composition, and its organization. Two-man "groups" can be devastating unless the individuals are known to be well suited. Admiral Byrd has graphically detailed the potential difficulties with two men in isolation (in this case, at an advance base in the Antarctic):

It doesn't take two men long to find each other out. And, inevitably, this is what they do, whether they will it or not, if only because once the simple tasks of the day are finished there is little else to do but take each other's measure. Not deliberately. Not maliciously. But the time comes when one has nothing left to reveal to the other; when even his unformed thoughts can be anticipated, his pet ideas become meaningless drool, and the way he blows out a pressure lamp or drops his boots on the floor or eats his food becomes a rasping annoyance. And this could happen between the best of friends....

With larger crews a variety of individual reactions may be observed. Within days or weeks there are often signs of interpersonal frictions, such as irritability, uncooperativeness, minor acts of rudeness, and even hostility. At this point some crew members begin to withdraw from group involvement, a process sometimes referred to as cocooning. Many crew members are surprised to discover how lonely they feel, even though they are surrounded by others with the same experience. This phenomenon has been aptly dubbed "the lonely crowd."

As communication and other social interactions become reduced to a minimum, territoriality and privacy needs assume prominence. The claiming of objects and areas is a feature of all isolated groups. A poignant example is the case of two life-raft survivors, adrift for a month. One of the two survivors refused to give up his only flashlight, even when he became too weak to use it for signaling. Such instances of territoriality reflect an attempt to maintain some measure of privacy. To quote Admiral Byrd again:

> Even at Little America I knew of bunkmates who quit speaking because each suspected the other of inching his gear into the other's allotted space; and I knew of one who could not eat unless he could find a place in the mess hall out of sight of the Fletcherist who solemnly chewed his food twenty-eight times before swallowing... little things like that have the power to drive even disciplined men to the edge of insanity. During my first winter at Little America I walked for hours with a man who was on the verge of murder or suicide over imaginary persecutions by another man who had been his devoted friend. For there was no escape anywhere. You are hemmed in on every side by your own inadequacies and the crowding pressures of your associates. The ones who survive with a measure of happiness are those who can live profoundly off their intellectual resources....[10]

With so many stresses and so few opportunities for expression and release, it is not surprising that psychosomatic symptoms are common. Difficulties with sleep are widely cited, as are headaches and episodes of nausea. Irritability and depression are frequent. Occasionally there are near-psychotic episodes that create a tense atmosphere for the remainder of the crew. What is more common, and almost as stressful, is the tendency for people to resort to compulsive behavior. Compulsive acts (which in other circumstances would be dismissed as minor eccentricities) may be magnified into major annoyances for the remainder of the group.

A few other aspects of group behavior should be addressed, since ignoring them inevitably leads to avoidable and unnecessary conflicts and group stresses. First, it is vitally important that the goals of the voyage be clear to everyone at the outset. It is a crucial mistake to assume that the goals are either obvious or implicit in the participation of the voyage. Second, it is equally important that all roles be explicitly assigned, especially those of the leadership. The leadership should be formal and defined. This is also true of the decision-making process. The leadership will wish to retain decision-making for all matters affecting the safety of the crew and vessel, and this should be clearly stated. In other areas, group decision-making may be appropriate. These areas should also be explicitly defined. *The absence of explicit role definition inevitably leads to accusations and recriminations and is the bane of many a sailing cruise.*

What can a captain do to influence and improve group behavior among a sailing crew? Proper selection of crew members is an important first step. Just as in solitary confinement, various individuals adapt differently to group confinement. The best indicator of future success as a crew member is prior crew experience or other exposure to small groups. In addition, the three factors of *work motivation, emotional stability,* and *social compatibility* are helpful in assessment. Biographic data have not been consistent predictors and should not be relied upon. Anyone with inappropriate motivation (e.g., escaping marital conflict) should be scrupulously avoided.

Anything that relieves boredom and monotony aboard ship is to be welcomed. In addition, every shipboard confinement contains numerous minor annoyances that are collectively trying, including lack of water for washing up, crowding, extremes of temperature, humidity, noise, and limited toilet facilities. These annoyances should be minimized as much as possible. In this regard, food is consistently noted as a highly important aspect of confined living, probably because it is one of the few pleasures still available! This should be kept in mind when planning a long voyage.

THE PSYCHOLOGY OF DISASTER

Contrary to the popular mythology, most individuals confronted with disaster do not panic, act hysterically, or become frozen with fear! In fact, the majority of disaster victims can contribute at least something to their own welfare and that of their companions.

It should not surprise us, however, that individuals do react somewhat differently to the tremendous stress of disaster. These differences are due, in part, to the underlying personality of each victim, his cultural background, and the specific nature of the disaster. Nevertheless, the obvious patterns of response that have merged from the study of disaster victims overshadow the differences. Anyone responsible for the lives of others—and every captain of a vessel certainly is—should be able to recognize the three characteristic stages of response to disaster. These were first described 30 years ago and continue to be as useful today in understanding the psychology of disaster.

The first stage is the *period of impact,* which continues until the initial stresses of the disaster are no longer present. During this period about 10 to 25 percent of disaster victims remain "cool and collected." These people retain an awareness of the overall situation, can appraise its consequences, and can formulate a plan of action. These people become de facto leaders. They may or may not have been formal leaders during the predisaster phase. The second group, comprising as many as 75 percent of the surviving crew, displays what has been called the "normal" psychological reaction. These people act bewildered and often have a restricted field of attention, lack of emotion, and a reflexive, automatic behavioral response. The third group, 10 to 25 percent, displays the manifestly inappropriate responses we tend to associate with disaster—panic, paralyzing anxiety, hysterical outbursts, confusion, and the inability to accomplish anything.

Following the initial stresses, or after the individual has escaped them, there is a *period of recoil.* Survivors characteristically show a childlike, dependent attitude, a yearning for comfort, and a need to ventilate their feelings, even if the moment is not opportune.

In *Two Against Cape Horn* Hal Roth provides one of the best descriptions of these first two stages. During a storm at night off Cape Horn, the Roths' anchors fouled and their boat was driven ashore. They were accompanied on this leg of their journey by a photographer and his wife (referred to as Adam and Eve). The Roths had never sailed with the photographer, and they had only spent a few days sailing with his wife. Both were novices aboard ship. The following account reminds us that the psychological reaction to disaster is no respector of either size or sex.

I had been so busy thinking about the wreck that I hadn't paid much attention to Adam. Now, when I looked closely at him, my heart sank. He was shaking in his boots. His eyes had become slits and he was almost crying. Instead of looking at me when he spoke, Adam looked at the ground. During World War II and the Korean War, I had seen what fear could do to a man.

"The yacht is finished," he said. "We don't even have a radio. How much food is there? I want an inventory of the food right away. We must count the cans.''

"Water?" said Adam nervously. "How much is there? How many days will it last? How much can we have each day? Let's sound the tanks right away."

I tried to reassure him. "I think we can get the yacht off," I said. "We may have to work in the water a little. I have a thick rubber wet suit...."

"Work in the water?"

I saw that Adam was horrified. It was clear that he wanted nothing more to do with the yacht....

Then, while I worked inside to expose the hull damage, I asked Adam to take the dinghy and row out an anchor. The wind had dropped and the job was easy. I told him exactly what I wanted, but when I looked out later I saw he had put the anchor out to the south, not the west. A fifteen-minute job had taken two hours and instead of securing the anchor warp to the port bow cleat to help pull the yacht toward deep water, Adam had put the warp on the starboard stern cleat which meant that he was tying the yacht to land. Maybe on purpose. Poor Adam was wandering about in a daze.

We had thousands of feet of new 16-mm film and two cameras on board. "How about taking some footage of the wreck and what we're doing?" said Margaret to Adam during the afternoon. "After all, a photographer doesn't have this opportunity every day."

"You're entirely right," said Adam in his deep bass voice....

Adam talked eloquently but he took no photographs—then or in the days to follow. Later he climbed into the yacht where I was working. He was looking for something and began to pick up things from the high dry side and let them fall into the water on the low side of the saloon or galley. He took a large plastic jar with all my taps and dies and drills from a tool drawer that I had open. His eyes were searching for something else so he simply dropped these irreplaceable tools into the salt water. I gasped. I could hardly believe what I had seen. At first I was angry, but as I moved closer to shout at him I saw Adam's eyes were glazed and that he was breathing heavily. He was sick with fear and not in control of himself....

After a few days he entered the period of recoil:

Adam liked the camp but he still acted nervously. He slept at least ten hours a night and spent hours writing furiously in a notebook. We repeatedly asked him to use the movie cameras, but nothing happened.[11]

The third phase is known as the *posttraumatic period*. It is during this phase that the survivors may begin to experience symptoms of "post-traumatic stress disorder." The survivor may continually ruminate about the event. Daydreams, nightmares, and even flashbacks may occur during which the event is relived. Anger is common during this period, occasionally associated with explosive behavior. Often, however, anger is directed in inappropriate and irrational ways. This phenomenon may produce "scapegoating," directed toward either groups or individuals. Survivor guilt is another frequent emotional reaction. Some survivors ruminate about whether they did enough in their rescue attempt. Others feel guilty simply because they survived while others, felt to be more deserving, perished. This kind of response can be emotionally devastating.

Emotional detachment is especially frequent. In addition, there may be a mixture of anxiety and depression. Other symptoms include an increased startle response, poor memory, and difficulty falling asleep.

ACCIDENTS

Accidents represent the fourth leading cause of death in the United States, after heart disease, cancer, and stroke. For those younger than 44, accidents are the *leading* cause of death. Probably no group is more sensitized to the problem of accidents than is the boating community. The ultimate goal, of course, is accident prevention. However, we are somewhat hampered in achieving this goal by the traditional concept of the accident. To many people, an accident implies that something *undesirable* has occurred that was *unanticipated* and thus probably *uncontrollable*—in other words, an unpredictable encounter between man and his environment. Sometimes this concept is useful. The tourist who was struck and killed by a cable while walking across the Brooklyn Bridge was certainly the victim of an accident. He had no way to anticipate and hence protect himself. It was a freak occurrence.

But many incidents that we label as accidents probably can be anticipated. For example, if in haste we overload a dinghy (to avoid making two trips) and it subsequently overturns, is that an accident? Many would probably label it an unfortunate boating accident, but what would be the implication of such a phrase? Obviously, someone should have anticipated the potential for danger. Instead, there was a serious mistake in judgment. To label it an accident, however, would be in a very real sense to abdicate responsibility: "It could have happened to anybody," "Just one of those things," and so forth.

> If we label all of life's unpleasant surprises as accidents, then we come to perceive ourselves as the playthings of fate and we cultivate a philosophy of carelessness and irresponsibility. On the other hand, if we look for causes and hold ourselves accountable for the mishaps in our lives, we become people of resource and confidence, increasingly able to control the direction of events. If these conclusions are as true as I think they are, it matters very much how we define the word accident.[12]

Some social scientists would go further:

> The term "accident"... refers to a makeshift concept with a hodgepodge of legal, medical, and statistical overtones.... Defined as a harmful encounter with the environment, a danger not averted, an accident is...subject to prediction and control. But defined as an unpredictable event, it is by definition uncontrollable.... The word should be discarded in scientific discussion.[13]

Not only is there a problem with definition, but, in addition, many otherwise intelligent people have developed a peculiar defeatist attitude toward accidents. Six of the most popular fallacious attitudes include:

1. The "other fellow" concept, whereby it is assumed that accidents happen to other people but won't happen to you.
2. The "your number's up" concept, whereby it is assumed that "when your number is up," you will get hurt and there is nothing you can do about it.
3. The "law of averages" concept, whereby accidents and injuries are shrugged off as due to inevitable statistical laws.
4. The "price of progress" concept, whereby accidents are rationalized as the inevitable price of scientific advancement.
5. The "spirit of '76" concept, whereby living dangerously is glorified and safety measures are regarded as for sissies.
6. The "act of God" concept, whereby accidents are seen as divinely caused—for punishment or for some purpose unknown to us.[14]

Are there people who are truly "accident-prone," and is there any way to identify them? This is a controversial area at the present time. Although several authors in the past have gone so far as to list personality traits characteristic of the accident-prone individual, most current authorities question the validity of such descriptions. Some have gone further and have called into question the concept that there are people who perpetually have a high "accident attraction" or "accident magnetism." In fact, the few studies that support the concept of the accident-prone individual were performed in the early part of this century and for the most part have not been duplicated.

Nevertheless, there probably is a small group of people with psychological conflicts associated with an increased incidence of accidents. Psychiatrists have long recognized that unresolved guilt may prompt self-punishing, masochistic behavior or excessive risk-taking, either of which may lead to accidents. Accidents may also be an unconscious means for the sailor to extricate himself from a threatening situation. If that seems farfetched, consider the psychological reaction of one of the OSTAR racers (a naval officer who did very well in the race): "I'd have taken any excuse to give up. *Wild Rocket* [a 63-foot schooner in the race]—lucky chap to have his sails blow out close to port."[15]

The current concept in recent studies of accidents is that both the *situation* and the *individual* must be considered. Certain endeavors such as boating are more dangerous and unpredictable than others. It should come as no surprise that these activities are associated with a high accident rate. At the same time, certain psychological and physical problems in the sailor increase his accident-proneness. In the short term, personal crises (worry, grief) and temporary physical conditions (fatigue, weakness following an illness) may temporarily produce an accident-prone individual. Over the long term, chronic psychological disorders (anxiety, depression) as well as physical limitations (poor eyesight, tremor) may impair a sailor's ability to do a specific job safely. Thus, accident-proneness does exist—for some people for brief periods of time, whereas for others for longer periods of time—but it should be considered in the context of the situation. Certainly, it would be reasonable to avoid taking on as crew anyone who is continually involved in boating accidents!

Finally, it is appropriate that the final chapter should address the problem of accidents, since the purpose of this book is, in a very real sense, accident prevention. For the sailor, especially, to be forewarned is to be forearmed. If the sailor understands how the human body functions in a marine environment, he is often able to anticipate potential accidents or difficulties and to avoid them. But this book is intended to be more than merely a guide to accident prevention on the water. It also attempts to provide the sailor with the knowledge he needs to promote health and happiness for himself and his crew. This is not an easy task. I know of no other activity that so challenges both our mental and physical abilities as does sailing. Enjoyable and successful sailing truly requires a sound mind in a sound body!

NOTES

1. Woodburn Heron, "The Pathology of Boredom," *Scientific American* 196 (1957):52-56.
2. The monotonous environment of many hospital intensive-care units is conducive to perceptual deprivation. The meaningless hum of life-sustaining equipment and an unchanging visual environment in which it may not be possible to distinguish night from day characterize these units.

3. Glin Bennet, "Medical and Psychological Problems in the 1972 Singlehanded Transatlantic Yacht Race," *Lancet* 2 (1973): 747-754.

4. Glin Bennet, "The Challenge of the Mind," *Cruising World,* August 1982, pp. *A*36-41.

5. Joshua Slocum, *Sailing Alone Around the World* (New York: Scribner's, 1978), pp. 59-60.

6. Bennet, "Medical and Psychological Problems," p.12.

7. E. C. B. Lee and K. Lee, *Safety and Survival at Sea* (New York: Norton, 1980), p. 177.

8. N. Tomalin and R. Hall, *The Strange Last Voyage of Donald Crowhurst* (Sevenoaks: Hodder & Stoughton, and New York: Stein and Day, 1970), pp. 248, 259, 274.

9. This is not to imply that there is nothing noteworthy about Crowhurst's psychological state. Both his egomania and his attempt at deception suggest some element of personality disorder. However, these personality traits are not by themselves associated with psychotic breakdowns.

10. Seward Smith, "Studies of Small Groups in Confinement," in *Sensory Deprivation: Fifteen Years of Research,* edited by J. P. Zubeck (New York: Appleton-Century-Crofts, 1969), p. 381.

11. Hal Roth, *Two Against Cape Horn* (New York: Norton, 1978), pp. 187-191.

12. J. J. Brownfain, "When Is an Accident Not an Accident," *Journal of the American Society of Safety Engineers,* September 1962, p. 20.

13. J. J. Gibson, "The Contribution of Experimental Psychology to the Formulation of the Problem of Safety," in *Behavioral Approaches to Accident Research,* edited by H. H. Jacobs (New York: Association for Aid to Crippled Children, 1961), pp. 77-89.

14. C. E. Richardson, F. V. Hein, and D. L. Farnsworth, *Living* (Glenview, Illinois: Scott, Foresman, 1975), pp. 339-340.

15. Bennet, "Medical and Psychological Problems," p.13.

Appendix

COMMON DRUG EQUIVALENTS*

	U.S.	U.K.	Canada	Australia
acetaminophen	Tylenol, Datril	paracetamol	Tylenol, Dolamin	Ceetamol, Tempra
amantadine	Symmetrel	Symmetrel	Symmetrel	Symmetrel
amitriptyline	Elavil	Elavil	Elavil	Elavil, Saroten
amoxapine	Asendin	Asendin	Asendin	Asendin
benztropine	Cogentin	Cogentin	Cogentin	Cogentin
biperiden	Akineton	Akineton	Akineton	Akineton
chlorothiazide	Diuril	Saluric	Diuril	Chlotride, Azide
chlorpromazine	Thorazine	Largactil	Largactil	Largactil
cyclizine	Marezine	Marzine	Marzine	Marzine
demeclocycline	Declomycin	Ledermycin	Declomycin	Ledermycin
desipramine	Norpramin	Pertofran	Norpramin	Pertofran
dextroamphetamine	Dexedrine	Dexedrine	Dexedrine	
dimenhydrinate	Dramamine	Dramamine	Dramamine, Nauseatol	Dramamine, Andrumin
diphenhydramine	Benadryl	Benadryl	Benadryl	Benadryl
doxepin	Sinequan	Sinequan	Sinequan	Sinequan
doxycycline	Vibramycin	Vibramycin	Vibramycin	Vibramycin
ephedrine	ephedrine	ephedrine	ephedrine	ephedrine
fluphenazine	Prolixin	Moditen	Moditen	Anatensol
furosemide	Lasix	Lasix	Lasix	Lasix
griseofulvin	Fulvicin, Grisactin	Fulcin, Grisovin	Fulvicin	Griseostatin
haldoperidol	Haldol	Haldol	Haldol	Serenace
hydrochlorothiazide	Hydrodiuril	Esidrex	Esidrex, Diuchlor H.	Esidrex, Dichlotride
hydroxyzine	Vistaril	Atarax	Atarax	Atarax
imipramine	Tofranil	Tofranil	Tofranil	Tofranil
isocarboxazid	Marplan	Marplan	Marplan	Marplan

Drugs are often marketed under a number of different proprietary names within each country. Only the most common examples are provided. If in doubt, use generic names, since they are usually similar from country to country.

246

	U.S.	U.K.	Canada	Australia
lithium	Eskalith, Lithobid	Camcolit, Liskonum	Carbolith, Lithane	Camcolit, Priadel
loxapine	Loxitane		Loxapac	Loxapac
maprotiline	Ludiomil	Ludiomil	Ludiomil	Ludiomil
meclizine	Antivert, Bonine	Meclozine, Ancoloxin	Bonamine	Ancolan
molindone	Moban			
nalidixic acid	NegGram	Mictral	NegGram	NegGram
nortriptyline	Aventyl	Aventyl	Aventyl	Aventyl
oxytetracycline	Terramycin	Terramycin	Terramycin	Terramycin
pargyline	Eutonyl	Eutonyl		
perphenazine	Trilafon	Fentazin	Trilafon	Trilafon
phenelzine	Nardil	Nardil	Nardil	Nardil
prednisone	Deltasone	Deltacortone	Deltasone	Deltasone
prochlorperazine	Compazine	Stemetil	Stemetil	Stemetil, Compazine
promazine	Sparine	Sparine	Sparine	Sparine
promethazine	Phenergan	Phenergan	Phenergan	Phenergan
protriptyline	Vivactil	Concordin	Triptil	Concordin, Triptil
scopolamine	scopolamine	hyoscine	hyoscine	hyoscine
tetracycline	Achromycin	Achromycin	Achromycin	Achromycin
thioridazine	Mellaril	Mellaril	Mellaril	Mellaril
thiothixene	Navane		Navane	Navane
tranylcypromine	Parnate	Parnate	Parnate	Parnate
trifluoperazine	Stelazine	Stelazine	Stelazine	Stelazine
triflupromazine	Vesprin		Vesprin	
trihexyphenidyl	Artane	Artane	Artane	Artane

Index